> Practices are changed by changing ways in which they are understood.
>
> Carr, W., Kemmis, S. (1986: p 91)

Transformative Reflection for Practicing Physicians and Surgeons:

Reclaiming professionalism, wisdom and moral agency

Della Fish MA MEd PhD Dip Ed/PGCE FAcadMEd

Della Fish's early career as a teacher educator, her wide knowledge of English literature and her observation of hundreds of consultants teaching in the clinical setting, underpins her unique career as a postgraduate medical educator. Della has worked with almost every healthcare profession as a teacher and an examiner to raise standards in curriculum design and development and in the activities of teaching, learning and assessment for postgraduates in the clinical setting. Her seminal book, *Refocusing Postgraduate Medical Education: from the technical to the moral mode of practice*, was published in 2012. She has taught at Masters level in five universities and in 2015 she designed and led the development of the five new core curriculum booklets for doctors as supervisors that make up the series *Medical Supervision Matters*, being both the lead writer in the four main booklets, and editing the series along with Linda de Cossart and Tim Wright. Della Fish is a visiting professor at the University of Chester and from 2008, until its recent closure was an Adjunct Professor in the Education for Practice Institute at Charles Sturt University, Sydney Australia.

Linda de Cossart CBE ChM FRCS FAcadMEd

Linda de Cossart continues actively to promote her credo that we influence the quality of clinical practice by who we are, how we respond to our responsibilities as clinical practitioners and the efforts we make as clinical teachers in Postgraduate Medical Education. She was a consultant vascular surgeon at Chester for twenty-two years and Associate Postgraduate Dean in Merseyside.

As co-director of Ed4medprac Ltd she has published widely and taught nationally and internationally with Della. She is a visiting professor at the university of Chester and is a former vice-president of the Royal College of Surgeons of England and was awarded a CBE in the Queen's birthday honours in 2010 for services to medicine and healthcare.

Studies in Education for Medical Practice
Book Two

Transformative Reflection for Practicing Physicians and Surgeons:

Reclaiming professionalism, wisdom and moral agency

Linda de Cossart & Della Fish

First published by The Choir Press in
association with Aneumi Publications in 2020

Copyright © 2020 Linda de Cossart and Della Fish

All rights reserved. No part of this publication may be reproduced or transmitted in any form or by any means, electronic or mechanical including photocopying, recording or any information storage or retrieval system, without prior permission in writing from the publishers.

The right of Linda de Cossart and Della Fish to be identified as the author of this work has been asserted by [them] in accordance with the Copyright, Designs and Patents Act 1988

First published in the United Kingdom in 2020 by
The Choir Press in association with Aneumi Publications

ISBN 978-1-78963-034-3

The Choir Press is a trading name of Action Publishing Technology Ltd
Registered in England & Wales, 132 Bristol Road, Gloucester, GL1 5SR

Aneumi Publications
An imprint of ED4MEDPRAC Ltd
A Limited Company: Registration No: 05648049
The Lodge
Cranham Corner
Cranham
Gloucester, UK
GL4 8HB

email: via www.ed4medprac.co.uk

Cover design, artwork, layout and type set in Gill Sans by Zero21media
www.zero21media.co.uk

Contents

Figures and Tables — xi
Acknowledgements — xiii
Foreword — xv

Introduction to the book — 1
    The long term aim of this book: a radical proposal to restore the standing of professionals and the professions — 3
    Our immediate intentions — 4
    The structure of this book and its title — 5
    The readership — 6
    Endnote — 6

Part One Transformative Reflection: an overview — 7
Introduction to Part One — 8

1. A radical proposal and rationale for re-motivating professionals and the professions: the need for Transformative Reflection — 11
    Introduction — 11
    The signs and symptoms of dis-ease in the medical profession — 11
    The diagnoses and remedies for these problems in the medical profession — 16
    Our critique of a recent and significant published view of the professions — 18
    Transformative Reflection: our diagnosis and our rationale for this book — 21
    Endnote — 22

2. Reflection: the essential core of learning through practice — 23
    Introduction — 23
    Our educational philosophy — 23
    An overview of reflection on practice — 27
    Reflection for doctors — 33
    Endnote — 36

3. Historical perspectives: the development of ideas about reflection as a practice — 37
    Introduction — 37
    Key thinkers in the development of reflection on practice — 38
    The changing focus of reflection: four developmental stages — 44
    Endnote — 47

4. The Transformative Reflective Process revealed: a detailed Introduction — 49
    Introduction — 49

What TRP offers to doctors that previous reflective processes have failed to provide	49
The Principles and Components of TRP	51
Transformative Reflection: how the components interrelate	53
Our educational thinking now underpinning Transformative Reflection	54
The Narrative and Exploratory Invisibles	57
A short comment about each of our eight Invisibles	61
Endnote	64

Part Two Transformative Reflection: The process and methodology — 65

Introduction to Part Two — 67

5. Prioritising time, selecting the case and developing the bullet points — 69

Introduction	69
Prioritising time for learning this new activity	69
Wise case selection: being alert to the educational opportunities	70
The implications of writing digitally or by hand	71
Creating the Bullet Points	71
An example of a set of bullets	72
Endnote	73

6. Transformative Reflective Writing: Creating the doctor-centred narrative — 75

Introduction	75
Creating your narrative using The Narrative Invisibles and their Prompts	77
Refining Your First Draft	91
An example of Rainbow Writing by a consultant surgeon	95
Endnote	98

7. Interrogating your Case Narrative to explore your Clinical Decision Making and Professional Judgement — 99

Introduction	99
A *review* of your current narrative	99
Exploring your Professional Judgements and Clinical Decision Making	100
Assessing the quality of your Clinical Thinking	105
An Example of identifying Professional Judgements and Clinical Decisions	107
Endnote	114

8. Summarising the results of your efforts — 117

Introduction	117
The emergence of key insights and new understandings	117
Responding to Appraisal and the GMC requirements	118
Endnote and a caution	120

Part Three Preparing for and planning to teach Transformative Reflection — 121

Introduction to Part Three — 123

9. Preparing to teach your junior colleague to engage in transformative reflection: educational starting points — 125

- Introduction — 125
- Understanding how to work in the moral mode of educational practice — 126
- Starting with your learner: seeing them anew — 128
- The learner and the formal PGME curriculum — 131
- New roles for the teacher and learner — 132
- Understanding the role of talking and writing for learning — 134
- The importance of using assessment to nurture the learner — 136
- Endnote — 139

10. Practical help for teaching the Transformative Reflective Process: thinking like a teacher — 141

- Introduction — 141
- Why learn to engage in Transformative Reflection? — 142
- Planning an educationally worthwhile programme — 143
- A short introductory programme for those newly learning TRP — 144
- Planning a face-to-face learning event as part of the introductory programme — 147
- Planning for a learner experienced in the TRP — 152
- Some useful teaching strategies: Using talking and writing — 154
- Finally, some evaluative questions for teacher to ask self — 159
- Endnote — 160

Part Four Reaching for the Future — 161

Introduction to Part Four — 163

11. A wider perspective on the value and use of the Transformative Reflective Process: understanding others' thinking — 165

- Introduction — 165
- Physicians and surgeons understanding themselves: why and how? — 166
- Physicians and surgeons sharing their thinking with others: why and how? — 167
- The Vital need for Researching Reflective Practice as a means of developing Medical Practice — 171
- The implications for other professions beyond healthcare — 173
- Endnote — 173

12. Mind your heart! Considering Spiritual Perspectives in reviewing your chosen case — 175

- Introduction — 175
- Seeing with the heart not the head — 176

Aims and Intentions of this chapter	176
The structure of this chapter	178
Two key perspectives on wisdom	178
A brief contextual survey of some ideas and values that challenge our understanding of spirituality	182
A conversation exploring spiritual practice and spiritual wisdom	185
The wisdom of the heart: an heuristic for a new Invisible	191
Endnote	192

Appendix 193
Transformative Reflective Writing: An Example The case of cholesteatoma disease. 195

References 209

Index 223

Figures and Tables

Figures

1.4.1	Transformative Reflection for Doctors: How the components interrelate	53
1.4.2	Transformative Reflection: The Process	54
1.4.3	The Invisibles. their Heuristic and their Reflective Focus	58
1.4.4	Rainbow Writing Colours	64
2.5.1	Bullet points of a consultant case	72
2.6.1	Rainbow Writing Colours for building the narrative	76
2.6.2	The Context Heuristic	78
2.6.3	The Iceberg Heuristic	80
2.6.4	The Extended/Restricted Professional Continuum Heuristic	82
2.6.5	The Extended/Restricted Professional Grid	82
2.6.6	The Knowledge Heuristic	86
2.6.7	The Therapeutic Relationship Heuristic	88
2.6.8	The Wider-Perspective Heuristic	90
2.7.1	The Clinical Thinking Pathway (CTP) and the Influences during treatment	101
2.7.2	The Professional Judgement Heuristic	102
2.7.3	The Clinical Decision making Heuristic	104
2.7.4	Some explanation of the quality of the different forms of Professional Judgement	106
2.7.5	Pinpointing Professional Judgements and Clinical Decisions	108
2.7.6	The underpinning thinking to the Professional Judgements	111
2.7.7	The categorisation of the Clinical Thinking	112

2.8.2 A Summary of one consultant's use of the TRP	120
4.11.1 Results of brainstorming what managers think of doctors	169
4.12.1 The new heuristic: The wisdom of the heart	191

Tables

1.2.1 Some defining characteristics of reflective practice	33
1.4.1 The principles and components of TRP	51
2.8.1 How the Invisibles help your response to the four GMC Domains	118
3.10.1 A Programme of Learning Events for teaching TRP to new learners	148
3.10.2 Planning a Learning Event to be attended by both the teacher and the learner	150
4.11.1 Ideas for informing research into TRP and Appraisal	172

Acknowledgements

Our very special thanks go to **Professor Deborah Bowman MBE, FRSA,** British academic and Professor of Ethics and Law at St George's, who we were thrilled to have write an introduction to the book. She has done this during her already extremely busy life and we could not have asked for a more appropriate start. Thank you.

This is the second book in our series Studies in Education for Medical Practice. Its completion during the lockdown for the COVID 19 pandemic, comes after a long gestation. It has been made possible only by the generous and intelligent contributions of so many but particularly by **Professor Tim Wright, Lynne Thorogood, John Latham, Emma Woolley and Jamie Fanning**, all of whom have been part of the courses and workshops that we have run over the last ten years. We are particularly grateful for everyone who has attended the courses and workshops we have run and their comments and evaluations have, over the years, undoubtedly shaped our thinking. Thank you, all of you.

We are grateful for the careful reading and critiquing of the whole book but especially chapter twelve by **Professor Tim Wright**, Emeritus Professor of Education at Chester University his ideas have shaped the final draft and ensured a more rounded script. Thanks to him too for his statement on the back cover of the book.

Thank you **Dr John Launer**, Health Education England (and/or Tavistock Clinic), Programme Director for Educational Innovation, Health Education England, London, for your endorsement and encouragement.

We are grateful to **Miss Sinéad Davis FRCS**, Consultant Surgeon, whose ideas on how as a clinician, to 'do' Reflective Writing and how to explore the professional judgements and clinical thinking have influenced our work. We thank her particularly for her time and expertise in helping us create an example for this book. The clinical case we have constructed is a mixture of several patient cases. Any resemblance to a particular patient case is only by chance.

The final chapter of the book could not have happened without the willing and honest engagement in the idea by **Ann Hopper PhD** and **Monica Butler RSM**. Their commitment to the task has been unstinting. Their proof reading, critique and ideas, all given generously and in the spirit of growing and continuous searching, have been an inspiration.

Thank you **Renate Thomé** and **Stuart Warner** who, between wild swimming and walking, have read and re-read many drafts and offered wise and helpful comments and corrections.

We are grateful for the patience and expertise of **Miles Bailey**, of The Choir Press, Gloucester, and for his reassuring and helpful comments and encouragement. He has never once chided us for not getting scripts to him on time.

Without **Jo Richardson of Zero21media** and her consummate professionalism, technical expertise and artistic talent this book would never have been completed. Always available, patient and encouraging, she has ensured that the book design and preparation for publishing has been kept on track.

We cannot close without thanking the team that has brought Della to the point of being able to be part of the completion of the book. It has been a complicated five months. We thank especially the teams in emergency care, emergency admissions and Ward 9B at Gloucester Hospitals NHS Foundation Trust, especially **Dr Sam Guglani**, consultant oncologist. Thank you **Dr Matthew Heyward, GP and the community staff** who have been steering Della's care, and for the amazing *Home Instead* **Senior Care Team** who have quite literally got Della back on her feet. Thank you **Jean Corbett and office staff: and carers Teresa Whitehorn, Daisy Mahoney, Jude King, Zoe Pargeter, Anna Misiuk, Jeni Long, Stephanie Snell, Georgina Eastlake, Raffaelina Vevey, Tarryn Mcarthy and Amy Bartlett**.

Last, but by no means least, we thank **Evelyn Usher** for her patience, support, and rigorous proof reading which again has saved us from numerous errors, and especially for making lots of cups of tea.

Linda de Cossart CBE and Della Fish
July 2020

Foreword

Reflection has a mixed reputation in healthcare. I have experienced how mixed responses can be to reflection.

Twenty years ago, I led on the introduction of reflective practice to a graduate entry medical programme. That cohort of students - our first - comprised a highly motivated, thoughtful and engaged group of people, many of whom had given up the certainty of other careers to retrain as doctors. I knew them to be sensitive and considered. I had learned an enormous amount from their reflections and responses as they progressed through medical training and encountered the diversity of clinical experience on placements.

Nonetheless, when the formal structure of the 'reflective portfolio' was introduced, many of these naturally reflective people who had shown their capacity for reflective work in multiple ways already appeared to struggle. They spoke openly about their ambivalence and even resentment of the task. Some of them took against what they perceived as the artificiality of the portfolio with its broad, but predetermined themes as prompts. Others were keen to convey that they valued informal reflection, but that they disliked 'reflection on demand' as they characterised it. Some distinguished between the writing and the discussions with a portfolio reviewer, with the latter meetings recognised as developmental. Only a minority seemed to enjoy completing the reflective portfolio. That mix of feelings about reflection has been replicated over many more years and cohorts of both graduate and undergraduate medical students, even as the reflective work itself has evolved in response to evaluations and student feedback. Mixed feelings it seems remain the commonest reaction to reflection.

Those mixed feelings are also captured on social media when reflection is discussed among practising clinicians. Ambivalence, criticism and even hostility are commonplace. Yet, often many of those same practitioners regularly and informally share their thoughts and insightful reflections about their work and the nature of healthcare (subject, of course, to the expectations of confidentiality). The value of a colleague making a timely observation, offering support, demonstrating understanding and suggesting further resources to explore is evident daily on social media and in online networks. Reflection in action is available for all to see. At the same time, there are concerns about the burden of reflection and its place in progression and revalidation.

Why might reflection prompt such mixed emotions? Healthcare is a practical endeavour. From the earliest days of training, the emphasis is often on intervention and outcomes. The work is often fast-moving and happens under pressure: the pressure to be efficient, to be effective, to be professional, to be better and usually in a resource-constrained environment. Such a context may generate competing forces. First, the space and need to share the burden and to work through the complexity and uncertainty that imbue clinical practice. Second, there may be resentment that reflection is another task on a long 'to do list' which appears frustratingly manufactured in format and timeliness. Little wonder that ambivalence about reflection is frequently observed.

There may be other influences, perhaps less conscious, on the mixed emotions about reflection. When I was learning my craft in clinical ethics, I recall watching a senior and respected clinician telling his junior doctors "don't just do something, stand there". Their responses were revealing: uncertain smiles (was this a joke?), expressions of puzzlement and lingering silence. It wasn't merely a neat aphorism. It was revolutionary, subversive and central to why reflection is both essential and threatening. Those six words counter the 'act under pressure' narrative that can so dominate in healthcare. Those six words challenge perceptions of role and focus on outcome. They seek to create space for thought in an environment where moving from task to task in an effort to beat the clock is a daily experience. When he spoke those six words, that senior doctor was asking much of his eager students.

Those challenges to the norms of clinical practice and the predominant narratives about the same may simultaneously be welcomed and resisted. The imperative to think and the permission to pause before acting can be liberating and freeing; providing respite from the constant demands of 'doing' to 'think about doing'. Yet, it can also be threatening and disorienting. The invitation to explore beyond the professional carapace and to seek meaning in the myriad information, protocols, guidelines and structures that inform clinical work is powerful. To meet it takes courage.

For reflection, if it is to count, requires the courage to open well-developed defences, to recognise and to question choices hitherto unexamined, to interrogate our assumptions, to seek meaning in uncertainty and to tolerate discomfort. That is its transformative power; as the authors of this volume know well.

Power, especially the power to effect change, can be frightening and overwhelming as well as liberating. It is unsurprising that the notion of reflection prompts mixed feelings amongst students and clinicians. It is not something to be undertaken lightly. It is demanding and unsettling. It requires much of participants. It is potent. No wonder there is a risk that many seek to avoid, diminish or even mock the concept of reflection.

What's more, reflection is difficult to do. It demands commitment, courage and openness to often discomforting feelings. That difficulty leads to a conundrum in the way in which reflection is often presented. In attempts, well-meant, to make complex and deep work manageable, we focus on structures and rules for reflection itself. These are often thoughtfully-developed and well-intentioned framing devices such as forms, platforms and timescales, but perhaps they inadvertently create a sense of dissonance. The power of reflection is sensed and the attempts to tame it can appear incongruent or, worse, simplistic and patronising to those charged with completing 'reflective tasks' to accord with external demands. Participants sense the value and transformative potential of reflection whilst simultaneously being met with tick boxes, checklists and forms for signatures. The structures themselves undermine what is possible and set up an inevitably mixed response from those charged with 'doing reflection'.

It could though, as this book demonstrates, be otherwise. Reflection that is authentic, grounded, personal, responsive and meaningful builds on the transformative power rather than undercuts it. It creates trust in the process to grow. It facilitates development. It does not hurry or seek reflection to deadline or predetermined format. It is simultaneously containing and liberating. It allows meaning to flourish whilst acknowledging the inherently uncertain nature of healthcare work. It provides space for complexity and exploration without demanding simple solutions or premature conclusions.

This book models an approach to reflection that recognises and values its transformative power. It is a courageous volume. It does not dodge the challenges, complexities or uncertainties that inevitably imbue reflective work. Its authors are companions who walk alongside the reader who is curious about reflection, but they do not prescribe, preach or presume. It is a generous and inclusive book that meets its reader in a spirit of openness, curiosity and enquiry. If readers can meet the authors in a similar spirit, they will be changed. Indeed, to read this book is to engage in an act of transformative reflection. It is a gift to us all.

Deborah Bowman
May 2020

Introduction to this book

Introduction to this Book

> The long term aim of this book: a radical proposal to restore the standing of professionals and the professions
> Our immediate intentions
> The structure of this book and its title
> The readership
> Endnote

We believe this book offers a refined and definitive version of our thinking so far about reflection for doctors. But in the final section we do also indicate other possible ideas that may need to be developed further and researched into, in the future.

This book is specifically designed for and addressed to physicians and surgeons in hospital practice in the UK, who we shall now refer to as 'doctors', to enable them to explore and develop the quality of their own clinical thinking, which is at the heart of wise practice (Fish and de Cossart, 2007). We see it as a form of Reflective Practice and in principle, as appropriate to General Practitioners in the UK, and all other professionals, worldwide. We offer this now because we believe that its time has come.

Both the Academy of Medical Royal Colleges and the General Medical Council (GMC) (2018, 2019) strongly support Reflective Practice for doctors and the learning that can emerge from it. They recognise there is a range of ways that a doctor may choose in order to help them engage in reflection, the purpose being to learn from experience and to be able to demonstrate this learning. The ten key points offered by the GMC on being a Reflective Practitioner are very reassuring. Our disappointment with the advice to date, however, is the lack of focus of how reflection can enable a doctor to unpack their complex thinking, clinical decision making and professional judgements in relation to specific patient cases. Doing this would then increase their capacity and capability to develop their own practice, articulate to others what that practice is really about and increase everyone's understanding of the complexity of professional judgement in medical practice.

Reflection for doctors, we believe, is at its most educational when focused on cases from their real everyday practice in which they are intrinsically interested, and where their aim is to identify and appreciate their expertise. By recognising and understanding more fully the conscious and unconscious elements that drive their practice, they will have the essential basis to develop further, their expertise and wisdom.

We believe that what we offer in Transformative Reflection can radically enlighten a medical professional's understanding of themselves, their detailed thinking, and the nuances of their practice. The Transformative Reflective Process (TRP) can sharpen a doctor's acumen (their ability to make good judgements and take quick decisions) and enable them to articulate for themselves and develop further, the deepest elements of what characterises their practice, particularly their professional judgement and practical wisdom. In this sense it is therefore, truly educational. It also provides a means of sharing the complexity and special nature of medical practice with those both inside and outside medicine, who need to understand it better. It has the potential, we believe, when shared, to benefit society's understanding of what is involved *inside* medical practice and thus clarify what it is reasonable to expect from The NHS's human servants. We offer more ideas about how such sharing might be conceived and promoted, in the penultimate chapter of this book.

We have already taught the main components of Transformative Reflection (The Invisibles and Medical Reflective Writing) to about 500 senior doctors, and have extensive personal written evidence that all but one GP and one pathologist have evaluated it highly! We have distilled further our ways of learning and teaching this process. We have also promoted some research into how doctors have found the learning process and how they are using it. (Bullock et al., 2012; Thomé, 2012 and 2013.)

Indeed, we would argue that if doctors used this method with well-chosen cases and on a regular and intentional basis, their ability to make the tacit explicit within a patient case they have attended to, will become a habit of their practice and in time enable them to think more precisely and wisely during their practice.

This is essential because it will:

- improve their *detailed* understanding of their current practice and of themselves in that practice
- enable their thinking and being to be unearthed, critiqued and developed
- provide them with a means of being far more articulate about their expertise
- enable them to share this expertise far more broadly
- place persuasive evidence on record of their regular exploration and refinement of their practice
- be a means of contributing to legal cases crucial detailed information of a doctor's judgements and of the custom and practice of medicine
- if shared more widely, it should enable society, and individuals in it, to understand much better the complexity of doctors' decision making and their human and humane response to clinical events and patient cases.

Much of the supporting detail about reflection in Part One, Chapters One to Three, works at the level of principle and addresses practitioners across all kinds of professions. But all the detailed practical examples from there onwards are focused on medical practice. That said, many of the criticisms of the professional work of such doctors and of their contributions to society, are often levelled in language sometimes applied also to other professions. Further, many of the principles we propose for doctors to reassert their reputations, professionalism and moral agency, could be equally as re-motivating for all other professionals. Readers are therefore urged to start their entry into this book by reading this introduction followed by Chapter One, in order to understand how best they each might then use the chapters that follow.

The long-term aim of this book: a radical proposal to restore the standing of professionals and the professions

The long-term aim of this book is to re-motivate UK doctors particularly and professionals generally, to refocus how they see themselves and their practice and so recover their vocational view of their work as servants of society. We believe that the following seven-step pathway, will provide the means to this.

We invite professionals of all kinds, and particularly medical practitioners to:

i. re-discover their essential self, their humanity and their own personal commitment to professionalism

ii. explain more cogently and in better detail how they come to their key professional judgements and the role of their clinical decision making in validating this

iii. develop a new willingness to exercise their wisdom of mind and heart without fear, and not for their own gain

iv. recognise the need for a more contemplative approach to the thinking and decision making that inevitably impacts on the life of their patients and on themselves

v. find vivid ways to articulate, illustrate and provide evidence of these deeper matters, for themselves, their supporting systems and thus their profession

vi. use this evidence to call for a supporting system for their work — at all levels in institutions, in governing bodies and in government – that understands their purpose, shares their motivation and seeks to provide a more compassionate basis for their activities

vii. have the courage to lead their profession and the public they serve to understand the need to slough off the limited conditioning of the target-driven agenda, of seeing all motivation in negative, power-generated and greed-driven terms and to be open to the potential power of unconditional love.

Simply beginning on this pathway, at step one, by looking at case examples of one's own practice, will inevitably lead practitioners to an increased sense of self-worth and the ability to articulate to others the demands of complex practice and their capacities and expertise. These characteristics will emerge even from the most typical of cases a practitioner meets and this is where the reflective process should first begin before moving on to more complex and less straightforward examples.

Our aim to re-motivate professional colleagues in this way grows out of the way practitioners are currently labelled as belonging to a group which has lost its standing and become self-interested as opposed to serving their patients or clients and the public (see for example, Blond et al., 2015). In medical practitioners, the resulting sense of loss of dignity, self-worth and moral agency has become so devastating that many are expressing openly their mistrust in those in power and the young are now leaving their posts at a significant rate.

We work amongst doctors and surgeons in their clinical practice, helping them to reflect on their patient cases in ways they have found transformative of themselves as people, as well as of their practice. From extensive experience of this, we believe that much of the problem of disaffected doctors is the result of widespread misunderstanding of who doctors are as people and how they work, think and are motivated. We have seen at first-hand how both the current climate and the need of those in high places to exercise an apparently overweening desire for power and control over the professions, has all but stifled the creativity, imagination and humanity of those who serve us all. It seems that people at all levels of society are quick to lambaste doctors, driven by either fake news manufactured to sell papers, or half-truths resulting from not understanding what it is or is not fair to ask of doctors. Why should we expect perfection of these human beings, when we so readily excuse our own mistakes?

One of our goals in this book therefore, is to demonstrate how professionals through rigorous reflection on, and exploration of, their own practice, can reassert their own sense of purpose and become more aware of and articulate about their professional achievements, expertise and character – as evidence of their *bona fides*.

Recording these detailed case-reflections and explorations of the person, the knowledge and the clinical reasoning they brought to the care of a few cases selected for specific self-educational purposes, would create a substantial body of evidence that would re-establish the pattern of a professional's motivation. It would both drive them to practise well and to develop further, would improve the morale of the profession, would provide a sound evidential basis for gaining greater recognition of the contribution of the professions to the good of society, and would legitimate the demand for more support and less opprobrium from the public.

What we propose is not of course a quick-fix matter, but we believe that the whole enterprise can grow 'from the bottom up', as long as it is guided and supported by a fully educational and therefore developmental process. As we shall show in Part Two, this uses rigorous prompts and guides in a deeper educational way than is found in most approaches to reflective practice for doctors. This approach also takes account of humanity (however that might be defined) as a foundational element of the person we are. Although discussion of such matters as spiritualty is much avoided in the Western World, we show that this cannot be ignored in attending to the growth of our essential self, and as the basis for wise professional practice (and we would say of a good life). That is why we provide a final chapter in Part Four that explores spiritual wisdom and offers one further heuristic that might add to the exploration of the case narrative already created through rainbow writing, which uses a range of colours to indicate different perspectives on the case.

Our immediate intentions in this book

In order to fulfil these long-term aims, our more immediate intentions in this book are:

i. to offer the philosophy behind this book and to clarify its rationale via a review of the current context of professional work in the twenty-first century and some key current attitudes towards professionals today

ii. to provide arguments for why it is necessary to reassert these key professional qualities which we see as dormant within them, and to outline why Transformative Reflection on one's own personal professional practice is a means by which professionals can re-recognise in themselves and give evidence of these qualities

iii. to demonstrate the development of ideas about reflection, its purposes and uses within professional practice and show how our work contributes to that history and to establish the position of Transformative Reflection within these traditions

iv. to take the reader step-by-step through the processes of Transformative Reflection and to show how to produce written evidence of the insights that this creates for the individual involved and their readers

v. to help clinical teachers engage educationally with junior colleagues, at the appropriate level of cases, to introduce them to this whole process and their wider responsibilities in respect of the public

vi. to indicate how, when shared, this can contribute towards the reinstatement of the standing of professionals in the eyes of the public, the main professional bodies and the government

vii. to open up, in the final section of the book, some further avenues for exploration and research into Transformative Reflection.

We believe that the above broad aim and these seven intentions will resonate strongly with many readers.

The structure of this book and its title

There are four sections in this book which we describe below.

Part One, entitled 'Transformative Reflection: an overview', offers four chapters. Chapter One provides the background to the development of Transformative Reflection by exploring what we, and those doctors we work with, see as the current uncongenial context for professional work. It shows something of what *some* recent, passionate and wholly negative publicity about the work of some colleagues has wrought amongst professionals and offers arguments for reclaiming professionalism, wisdom, and the spirit of disinterested service for the good of individuals and society. We have also indicated that we see the best in doctors as able to be drawn out by educational processes and not as an agenda to be instilled from outside. Thus, we have attempted to fulfil the first two of our declared intentions.

Chapter Two provides a number of perspectives on reflection and indicates how reflection can be defined. Chapter Three illustrates the contribution of some key figures in the development of Reflective Practice and shows how our creation of Transformative Reflection fits into the history we have charted. Chapter Four offers an overview of the development of the elements of Transformative Reflection: The Invisibles and Medical Reflective Writing. By this means, Part One fulfils our third intention.

Part Two, entitled 'Transformative Reflection: The Process and Methodology', offers Chapters Five to Nine, providing the heart of the technical processes necessary for rigorous Transformative Reflection, and fulfils intention four.

Part Three, entitled 'Preparing for and Planning to teach Transformative Reflection', offers Chapters Nine and Ten which provide the educational approach to teaching junior colleagues this entire process — which should be started in Foundation Programmes (year one of the medical career). This completes intentions five and six.

Part Four, entitled 'Reaching for the Future' draws the book to a conclusion in Chapters Eleven and Twelve. Chapter Eleven, offers a vision of how we see the practical implications of taking a bottom-up approach to Transformative Reflection and how medical professionals might begin to educate the patients, managers and the broader public about how medicine really works and what is involved in serving individual patients to the best of their human ability. Chapter Twelve considers how bringing up spiritual perspectives to re-viewing a patient case, might offer a deeper set of questions to ask at the end of the reflective process. These two chapters complete the final intentions for the book.

The readership

We seek to address all doctors and to remind readers from professions other than medicine, to use those parts of the book that directly talk of professions generally and to infer and use the principles of procedure found in Parts Two and Three as best they fit their own specialties.

Endnote

We hope and even dare to believe that what we offer in this book about the current unacceptable view of professions and professionals, that has emerged at the end of the second decade of the twentieth century, will drive readers to: engage in Transformative Reflection; and be prepared to articulate far more about their expertise, firstly to themselves, secondly to colleagues (managerial and all healthcare professionals), and thirdly to patients, relatives and the public.

Part One

Transformative Reflection: an overview

Introduction to Part One

Part One offers the reader a context for why Transformative Reflection as described in this book is relevant to physicians and surgeons in developing wise practice. We believe from evidence of those who have engaged in using this process, that Transformative Reflection, is a means of better understanding oneself and one's practice as a professional. And as 'reflection on practice' (post practice), it will eventually become an invaluable habit of mind that drives and develops action *within practice*. It is seated generally within the traditions of Reflective Practice.

Chapter One contextualises why we think this process of learning is needed more than ever in the current context of medical practice in the UK. It attempts to diagnose the growing 'dis-ease' perceived by society about how doctors conduct themselves, by considering evidence of key symptoms and signs signalled from a variety of perspectives. Such evidence is itself problematic in that its motivations are not always clear and because it is inevitably focused on failures that patients and the public rightly find totally distressing. However, sometimes it seems to be implied that individual doctors have in some sense deliberately and carelessly jeopardised patient health when the reality is that systems and contexts in which they operate are far from supportive and they have in fact done their very best. This chapter then goes on to offer a range of proposed diagnoses towards remediating these matters and explains why we see Transformative Reflection as a healing option. It offers ideas on how professionals should refocus their view of themselves as professionals and should aim to share the complexities of medical practice with others within and outside the profession. It urges doctors to return to seeing the responsibilities of being a professional in the service of patients and the health of society.

Chapter Two explores our educational philosophy and the value of reflection as a worthwhile educational activity. It offers an overview of reflection generally, emphasising its educational importance today when doctors and those who teach them are spending fewer hours actually in practice and even fewer sharing together the subtleties and nuances of being a wise practitioner. It emphasises the need to make the most out of fewer experiences.

Chapter Three provides an overview of the development of reflection-on-practice (Schön). It sets out a critical historical review and follows this with details about reflection within healthcare and medical practice. It emphasises Reflective Practice as a practice in its own right and the need for rigor and discipline within this. It comments on the importance of both talking and writing reflectively and the transformative effect of intelligent reflection.

Chapter Four charts our extensive experience of exploring and creating a process where the focus of reflection for doctors is on the quality of their professional judgements and their underlying clinical reasoning leading to action. This is, as far as we are aware, the only process that has focused on doctors' specific needs, most reflection templates having been adopted from professions other than medicine. The development of our work, which we now call Transformative Reflection, offers a process that is centrally educational and conforms to the idea that a truly educational enterprise literally changes the learner in serious ways that deepen their self-understanding and appreciation of their expertise.

Chapter One

A radical proposal and rationale for re-motivating professionals and the professions: the need for Transformative Reflection

Introduction
The signs and symptoms of dis-ease in the medical profession
The diagnoses and remedies for these problems in the medical profession
Our critique of a recent and significant published view of the professions
Transformative Reflection: our diagnosis and our rationale for this book
Endnote

Introduction

This first chapter begins by providing a brief overview of a range of current perspectives, at the end of the second decade of the twentieth century, that are seriously critical of medical practice and of the conduct and character of doctors. We seat our ideas on Transformative Reflection within the need to respond to these serious concerns. We offer these perspectives under the headings: the signs and symptoms of the dis-ease of the medical profession; diagnosis; and currently proposed remedies. This is followed by a detailed critique of one example of a very recent critical report on the state of trust between doctors and society. We then offer our own sense of the state of medical practice as drawn from our own shared and extensive experience of working in postgraduate medical education. This chapter ends with our proposals that Transformative Reflection can be doctors' key means of becoming equipped to articulate to those who misunderstand them: who they are, how they think and what they do.

The signs and symptoms of dis-ease in the medical profession: five viewpoints

We identify the signs and symptoms (the evidence) of the current 'dis-eased' state of medicine and of the medical profession as articulated from the viewpoints of five different groups. Their offerings are often presented as objective facts but are driven by their own — usually unacknowledged — agendas. Thus, the evidence (signs and symptoms) of dis-ease in the practice of medicine is articulated by:
  i. some understandably distraught patients whose cases were compromised, together with their relatives and friends
  ii. the regulators and controllers of medical practice and the medical profession
  iii. the media of all kinds and the fluctuating views of society at large
  iv. some lawyers and ethicists who inevitably seek a dualistic (or black and white

view), rather than a deliberative moral view which seeks not compromise but a unitive view
v. the doctors themselves.

The first four viewpoints

The first four of these viewpoints seem to highlight key evidence of the apparent failure in individual doctors, and often imply carelessness or at least some failure of a doctor to 'get it right', which is often then generalised immediately to the unsatisfactory state of the whole profession. We believe that whilst some doctors do indeed deserve to be punished and/or struck off and that such cases do escalate a desire for justice and redress, this growing immediate urge to blame and seek 'revenge' partly springs from the false assumptions prevalent in society which expects doctors to be perfect human-beings. We shall comment on the doctors' own viewpoints later.

The main complaints from some patients, regulators and controllers of medical practice, the media, and some lawyers and ethicists, unless very clear-cut (which few actually are), seem to be based on myths, impressions and negative agendas, as the following *sample* accusations indicate.

- Patient cases that have gone wrong are the doctor or doctors' ultimate fault and responsibility, irrespective of the fact that many such failures arise from a concatenation of circumstances in the system as well, perhaps, as unbelievable pressures at individual level.

- Such cases provide irrefutable evidence of the generally poor preparation and education of doctors.

- Beneath the publicly revealed tragic cases that clearly contained many mistakes, and the few psychologically sick doctors who were indeed mass murderers, there grows the society-wide but false impression of an unacknowledged underworld of carelessness, culpability, arrogant ignorance and even evil on the part of some doctors and a suspicion that this is true of most of them.

- The mismanagement of cases, and other ills and evils, prompts the immediate blame of a doctor or doctors, often followed swiftly by a call for retribution. This encourages the regulators of professional conduct to find a scape-goat, the lawyers to seek to convict, and the law and the controllers, including politicians, to fix punishment – which may ruin the career of the individual, labelling them as 'wrong-doers'. Unfortunately, this suggests that most medical errors or undesirable outcomes were avoidable or even deliberate, when many were probably more about a misjudgement made in the messy and complex environment that is clinical practice.

- Mass public demonstrations in support of the relatives of tragic cases, irrespective of what has gone wrong, suggest the large-scale loss of public support for doctors (with rarely an investigation into whether or not these large demonstrations have actually been an expression of sympathy for the bereaved or in fact orchestrated for political ends).

- The perception is thus crystallised of a general malaise and a siege mentality on the part of doctors and their professional bodies.

- An overwhelming sense prevails that doctors can make mistakes and that now we know this, they can no longer to be trusted, though this goes against even recent surveys in which doctors are still held as the most trusted of all professionals.

- As a consequence of all that has gone wrong, there is an apparent loss of direction of professionalism, and a change in society's attitudes to it.

- In the second decade of the twenty-first century there has been a dramatic leakage of doctors from their posts in the UK to other countries where many then settle.

Some of these ideas seem to be driven by jealousy about the status of doctors, and the attitude that any mistakes in medical practice deserve an individual to be characterised as a failure. A sickening example of this (both for the patient's relatives and for doctors) is the Bawa-Garba case, where the doctor's conviction for gross negligence has rocked medicine, and which on further investigation was seen more as a systemic issue of failure, over which individual doctors have only so much power. It is interesting to note too, that the fear of a law-court's abuse of reflective writing, which spread amongst doctors and made them (for a while) doubt the importance of reflection, was the result of seriously false news about the first trial.

It is interesting to note too, that all the above views are articulated by those who work outside the medical profession. It is safe to say that very few, if any, of these:

- has any knowledge of, let alone expertise in, medical practice

- understands the hugely complex and pressurised context within which doctors work

- knows about the traditions, and customs and practices that shape what doctors do and say and the meaning of this in context*.

- is privy to how doctors think and feel about the patients they care for

- recognises that how doctors appear visibly and publicly - to patients, to relatives, in legal contexts, or when speaking to the press or public - is only part of how they conduct themselves as a whole in their work setting, as driven by their personal feelings, values and beliefs.

* For example in the Bawa Gaba trial, a barrister accused her of not asking her supervisor to review the patient when she had actually reported all the alarming medical details to him, such that the tacit rule in practice meant that he should have checked that patient out. But the barrister did not understand that, and the damage of his accusation was done because the defendant did not fight back.

Much of the truncated information that is offered through these different viewpoints is often provided in sound-bites crafted to catch the attention of those who sell news, or by those who seek to keep the public informed, to impress fellow members of major controlling bodies, to demonstrate their finesse in ethical argument, or to convince a court of law. And some of it is generalised smearing of the whole medical profession, based on evidence from a very few high-drama cases that are serious and utterly distressing in themselves but which do not represent how the vast majority of doctors conduct themselves.

A fifth viewpoint: from inside medical practice

Why then, in response to all this opprobrium, have the doctors said very little about and demonstrated publicly only occasionally against, what is happening to medical practice? We firmly believe that it is because by and large, as members of a profession, doctors are still dedicated to the best care of patients, and beyond this, the ultimate good of society. Thus, they have mainly accepted what they have been asked to do in the name of better care for patients, and 'are getting on with it'. Further, being short-staffed in most departments in most hospitals, and needing to take on that work as their own, for the sake of patients, they have had little time to give to setting out their arguments. Also, mostly not being 'political animals', they have not been very good at constructing and presenting logical arguments for political purposes.

What follows — as a view from inside medical practice — is our own understandings of the symptoms of dis-ease within the medical profession, an agenda, derived from close work with doctors in the practice setting for many years. Linda gave a career's worth of work as a hospital surgeon, and together we now work with doctors to try to help them improve the education of their junior colleagues as a means to enhance patient care. Our agenda in this chapter is not either to be defensive of doctors or apologetic for them. We are well appraised of their human frailties and our own. We simply offer our professional impressions.

Together, we have concluded over the last fourteen years that the state of medical practice and postgraduate medical education has become more and more dire. During that time, we have (together and separately) been warning about the damage being done by over-control and regulation as well as narrow-minded management and the uncongenial context for recruitment as set by the regulators and controllers. This has incrementally eroded the way doctors both now see themselves and present themselves to their patients and society. As early as 2005 we wrote that because the political climate was becoming more controlling:

> highly motivated trainees and consultant teachers will be thoroughly demoralised if they do not take stock of their position in this changing world. (de Cossart and Fish, 2005:14)

We saw *Modernising Medical Careers* (MMC) as a prime mover in this change for the worse, and as a profound mistake with far-reaching consequences. Introduced in 2005 it was a new system for regulating postgraduate medical education, and thus the whole thrust of medical practice. It was negotiated between the medical professions and government with the specific aim of training doctors faster in preparation for the consequences of the European Working Time Directive. MMC is still the basis out of which the current system of medical practice and postgraduate medical education has grown. Della warned of its dangers in 2012, arguing that:

> both medicine and education have been re-packaged by MMC as purely technical practices in which we have lost sight of the creativity, sensitivity, flexibility and courage to produce personal rather than protocol-driven decisions and solutions which professional practices will always require. In short, both consumers and practitioners appear to have lost sight of the fact that professional practices like medicine and education require professionals to operate in both the moral as well as the technical mode of practice, where there are moral imperatives to find innovative and more broadly insightful solutions to technical problems.

She added:

> Indeed, professions have become so rigidly bound by regulation and the threat of litigation that many members have adopted a learnt helplessness in the face of 'the rules', expect to look outside themselves in order to be told what to do, and then accept and thus bow to the conditions that apparently make the problem insoluble beyond a little technical tinkering round the edges. Thus, we all forget that the whole point of being a professional is that there are serious responsibilities to take on some agency of our own in shaping our practice, and that a doctor's judgement about a way forward in a context-specific instance may well mean that they need to go beyond the surface and the protocol. (Fish, 2012a:3)

We must at this point make very clear that we were not the only ones concerned about professionalism. Indeed, it has been a recurring topic over at least the last twenty-five years. The key writers have included, Freidson, (1994 and 2001); Irvine, (2003, 2018); Marcotte, et al. (2020); Pereira Grey, (2000); Royal College of Physicians, (2005) and Southern and Braithwaite, (1998). We ourselves have also published on this topic: de Cossart and Fish, (2002, 2006, 2013); Fish and de Cossart, (2018); Fish and Higgs, (2007).

From our view point the symptoms of the dis-ease of medicine, from within the medical profession are that:

- there has been too much over control at macro and micro levels of medical practice

- there has been too much outside interference in matters that are the proper province of the profession itself

- the role of PGME has not been well explored with the needs of those senior practitioners in mind, who, as well as their clinical duties, have to engage in serious and complex teaching without more than a two-day course on training to prepare them and with little respect given to this vital role in patient care

- there have been too many rules and protocols about what doctors should do in specific situations, and too little understanding of the complexity of the professional judgements and clinical decisions that cannot be avoided and are not amenable to formulaic means laid down by writers who were never in the specific situation

- views about professionalism have changed and there is a gap between how doctors see their professionalism as members of a long extant and very respected profession, and how society treats anyone who claims to be a professional.

These five viewpoints then offer serious but diverging signs and evidence of what is amiss in medical practice and the medical profession.

The diagnoses and remedies for these problems in the medical profession

As we shall show here, the evidence of dis-ease as seen from outside medical practice leads to one set of diagnoses, while that seen from within medicine comes to a different conclusion.

The diagnoses as seen by those outside medical practice

The following two diagnoses emerge as central.

i. 'Many' individual practitioners are incompetent or irresponsible, or lacking in professionalism and the profession has failed adequately to regulate itself.

ii. What society needs is the reshaping of the whole enterprise of healthcare.

The diagnosis from within medical practice

This, of course, conveniently ignores the fact that the human tragedies that do occur (and which are a very small proportion of the huge number of patients treated) are as gutting for doctors as for patients and their relatives, and are often not the avoidable mistakes they appear to be, but rather the results of a concatenation of unexpected circumstances with only milliseconds to think before action.

By contrast and not surprisingly, the diagnoses of the 'dis-ease' within medical practice, as made by doctors themselves in our hearing, pinpoint similar problems but place the blame in an opposite camp. They argue that:

- the whole system of medicine is over-controlled from the macro to the micro level of the organisations and institutions within which doctors work

- the problems arise from the over-control of professional practitioners (rules, regulations and protocols) set by outsiders to be used in contexts where professionals actually need flexibility, authority and their own agency to act for the best, for each patient

- society lacks clarity about, and serious understanding of, what they can expect about the conduct and professionalism of those who still attempt to serve the public as doctors.

The treatment offered from these two views

This all illustrates that the 'diagnosis' — and the associated treatment plans – emerge from two opposite positions. Unfortunately, the dualistic nature of these virtually opposing views about what is wrong with medical practice seem to have been ignored, and the opportunity for any rapprochement between the two sides and the chances of learning by both, have been entirely lost. The fact that both 'sides' have important contributions to make in ameliorating the situation has been overshadowed because the loudest voices and the most widely broadcast complaints leave no room for other views, especially since public opinion is often gullible and easily swayed. And so the voices of doctors seem to us to have been drowned out. The result is that the demand for gross over-regulation of the profession and the debilitating denigration of doctors' motives and abilities, has become distorted and generalised so that many doctors we have worked with have a deep sense of loss of the meaning of their professional position in society and their motives and beliefs.

This has, in our experience, damaged in many doctors their personal sense of value and their self-belief. The irony here is that at the same time, society is demanding more and more service from them with fewer and fewer staff and other resources. It seems to us that more energy is expended by all involved in pinpointing the negative factors at play in the current state of medical practice, than is spent in trying to find better ways forward.

Currently then, the required treatment for all these woes seems to be greater control of the profession and of professional practice and the consequent lessening of the meaning of professionalism and what it is to be a professional who seeks the good of individuals and society. It thus seems that society is going to look to over-scrutinise the whole profession and use punishment as the major antidote to the failures of the few.

As we shall show shortly, we believe that the better way forward may be for doctors themselves to become more pro-active in reminding the public of:

- who they are
- what they do
- what their professionalism really consists of.

Before this, however, we review a significant recent report that offers some interesting thoughts on professionalism and how the public and the whole medical profession needs to review their understanding of what it is to be a professional.

Our critique of a recent and significant published view of the professions

In 2015, The ResPublica Trust (an independent and non-partisan think tank) published an important report: *In Professions We Trust*. (Blond et al., 2015). This Trust was spurred on and helped by staff at Birmingham University's Jubilee Centre for Character and Virtues (an educational institution with a strong agenda about the importance in all walks of life of character and virtue, as drawn from Aristotle's writings). The publication speaks of professions generally, but focuses on Medicine, Teaching and Law in particular. It offers an overview of its interpretation of the problem gap between society's perceptions of what it needs from doctors and what doctors themselves now offer society, and it makes recommendations for ways forward.

The Report's diagnosis does not, in our view, take account of all the symptoms (all the influences on current professional practice) and has an agenda that is not entirely independent. Particularly, it seems to hold doctors especially responsible for the gap between them and society, where it might reasonably have argued more strongly that there were other contributing factors like over-regulation at all levels from individual NHS organisations, through to national government and its agencies (for example, the Care Quality Commission). The industrial model of professional practice now rigidly links funding to control at macro and micro level and sets rules and protocols and thus (as far as possible and far further than is wise) removes professional judgement from the core of practice, leaving little agency to those on the ground.

Further in making its points and leading up to its recommendations, the report also ignores some of the more encouraging evidence of Healthcare practitioners (though not specifically doctors), attempting to maintain their own humanity despite the target-driven requirements upon them, and some members of the public too have raised their voices in opposition to the current culture across healthcare as set by the controlling agenda of the government. See for example, O'Neill (2002) Pollock (2004); Iliffe (2008); Seddon (2008); and Seldon (2009).

However, Blond et al. do usefully pinpoint the increasing ills of professional practice, as evidenced by The Francis Report (Francis, 2013), and a number of well publicised legal cases. Disastrous as they are, these events constitute a small number of cases compared with the many successes of everyday practice, but they are persuasively used in the Report to demonstrate 'a rupture of trust', between society and the professions where the link between them has 'already broken or is close to breaking'. This is seen as because 'the notion of a profession as of 'something which encompasses and adds to the public good' has disappeared', (2015:2). It implies, but does not state that it is, as we have been led to think by the media, the fault of the doctors. But there are probably three sides to this whole story: the doctors'; the institutions' (local and national); and the media's slant, designed to sell newspapers and capture television viewers.

Thus, there is no arguing against the fact that there is an increasing gap of trust between medical practitioners on one side and their patients and the public on the other. Given this diagnosis of the ills in medical practice, The Report, in its treatment plan, seems to bring to its thinking a particular lens, derived more from the work and agenda of the Jubilee Centre than from a deep understanding of postgraduate medical practice and of the education for it. The Jubilee Centre sees Aristotelian virtues and their goal of *eudemonia* (human flourishing) defined as unquestionably *the* key to 'human good'. However, such good or well-being, in which human flourishing occurs across a lifetime, might be based on other views about what might drive our conduct even beyond the exercise of moral virtue, practical wisdom, and rationality, as characterised by Aristotle. For example, a life with an acknowledged spiritual foundation would have a different view of service from others, motives for action and even the influences on professional judgement (as of the heart as well as the head). In fact, the report seems unaware of the expertise and humanity that doctors do bring to their practice and ignores the spiritual dimension that is often tacit in their conduct (see Chapter Twelve).

Further, in seeming to believe that virtue can be 'embedded' and 'instilled' into people rather than drawn out from them, The Report offers a somewhat naïve view of education. It also, unwisely, either dismisses or misunderstands the part that reflection can play in improving professional practice, arguing instead for:

> a systematic investment in examining professional life. This is distinct from reflective practice in that it involves a commitment to learning and changing otherwise referred to as 'reflexive critique'. This means that leading a virtuous professional life demands a commitment to examining and re-examining consciously professional life. (Blond et al. 2015: p.26.)

The irony here is that The Report dismisses Reflective Practice, replacing it with the term 'reflexive critique', which is commonly associated only with what might be called 'narrative reflection' as used in much of healthcare outside medicine. Narrative reflection prompts only surface changes in behaviour, unlike Transformative Reflection as offered in this book, which explores practice in depth with all its underlying moral obligations and complex expertise and ability to transform doctors and their practice.

It seems therefore that The Report's overview of the decline of professionalism is strikingly expressed and deserves serious critical attention. For example, it reminds us that originally professions were 'moral communities based upon shared expertise and occupational membership' and that: 'it was commonly held that the professions were both moral and technical orders that militated against both self-serving individualism and collectivist state' (Blond et al., 2015: 2). The Report implies that moral awareness is entirely missing in current medical practice, but our experience does not support such a negative view. Further, Transformative Reflection is precisely about heightening the awareness of doctors' moral agency.

Such over-generalisation is also true of the Executive Summary of The Report which offers its key critique thus:

> ... in recent times professions have come to be seen as self-serving interest groups propagating their own agenda and interests. They have increasingly come to be regarded as hostile to newcomers or challenges and uncaring about those whom they served .... During the 1960s they were seen as culturally elite and distant .... [later] ... they were deemed to have been captured by the producer interest – creating labour market shelters that did not serve the general welfare. (Blond et al., 2015: 3.)

It may be true that some doctors have 'lost sight of their necessary connection to the wider public good', and favoured the commodification view of practice in which they consider only the external goods to the point that there has been some fundamental disconnection between the internal goods of the profession and their external *raison d'être* to serve the public (Blond et al., 2015:3). But again this is patently not the case in most medical practice as we see it. We do not find (and the report offers no hard evidence for the idea) that those inside medicine amongst other professions are 'being oriented towards ways of working that conspire against noble understandings of what it means to be a professional, which is what the public wants and needs'. Indeed, any such orientation comes from the controllers and regulators outside medicine, not from most doctors within it, who would wish to challenge this.

Thus, we would argue that the ResPublica Report provides a very significant and succinct *contribution* to the expression of what is wrong with these professions (though it ignores the false messages and over-dramatisation of blame for which the media is largely responsible). Importantly, it adds weight to the need for something to be done about the relationship between the public and the professions. However, we find its overview of the problem somewhat narrow, and its conclusions and recommendations for a way forward, rather biased. Professionals alone are not responsible for the demise of their relationship with the public. However, they may be the only means of recovering their own reputation as an important basis for helping the public to recognise, that it is vital to re-establish 'a strong sense of partnership and mutual guardianship' between them and the professions.

Transformative Reflection: our diagnosis and our rationale for this book

Our interest here is not how these criticisms have developed, what are the rights and wrongs in the case, or whether individuals or systems are responsible for serious lapses. Our diagnosis is that one of the major problems at the heart of these complaints, (to which the rest of this book then provides a radical but essentially simple Treatment Plan) is that the writers of the Res-publica Report and those whose voices that are raised against doctors, do not understand in enough detail the complexity of medical practice and what lies beneath the surface of the visible elements of that practice. This is in major part because of the now contestable requirement on doctors to show no emotion, to hide their moral motivation and to deal with all eventualities with a cool imperturbability that avoids bringing the humanity of the doctor as a person to meet directly the patient as a person (Sokol, 2007). In the light of the current context of society and medical practice we believe that this idea needs serious revision.

Our treatment proposal is different from Res Publica's. It works 'bottom up' and is based on a belief in the humanity and spirituality as well as the technical expertise and broad intelligence of doctors. We argue that what is needed is a better understanding, first by practitioners and then by patients and the public, of the person the doctor brings to their practice and what drives their actions, judgements, reasoning, thoughts and feelings in a given case. The understanding of self and exploring one's being as a practitioner, is the way to developing confidence and the growing capacity for persistence in doing the right thing and for growing in wisdom as a professional.

This is why we suggest doctors might start by unpacking, in a disciplined and guided way, the implicit and tacit in a few of the individual clinical cases for which they are responsible. By this means they will uncover for themselves the detail of their expertise and evidence of the insights and educational development that arise from this, and become more articulate about it. As part of this they will learn to express more vociferously their own sense of vocation, which is currently not properly understood, along with their motivations, identity, professionalism and moral agency. In then leading other colleagues and gradually the public to understand better the complexities of practice and what they bring to that as human beings, they should in time bring about a far better appreciation in the public and even the media about who professionals are, what they bring to their practice, how they work in practice, what thinking and decision making drives this, and what wisdom (practical judgements and discernment) they generate as they work.

Endnote

We are persuaded that proper education is transformative, and that whatever is claimed to be education is not so unless it is has provoked serious and lasting change for the better. Our work with doctors has been dedicated to this end and this book offers an educational and well-tried way of supporting this.

Chapter Two

Reflection: the essential core of learning through practice

Introduction
Our educational philosophy
An overview of reflection
Reflection for doctors
Endnote

Introduction

This second chapter offers three main sections. The first provides a summary of our educational philosophy, out of which our ideas on reflection have been refined. The second offers an overview of reflection generally. The third focuses on reflection for doctors as specific to their unique role in healthcare.

We attend here to what, following Schön (1987), is generally called **reflection on practice.** This is a process which looks back on an event in our own professional practice with the intention of exploring it and learning from it. We believe that Schön's *'reflection-in-practice'*, where the practitioner is thinking during the heat of practice, develops best from an already well-refined ability to reflect retrospectively on practice (Schön, 1987, Chapter One).

Our educational philosophy

Education is itself a values-based concept, and therefore both problematic and not readily definable. However, there are key principles that 'educators' of all kinds would espouse in common. Indeed, in the 'conversations of mankind' about education that have taken place in the West, over at least the last 2,500 years, we find much that is held in common about what is involved in 'good' education, or as we would prefer to say: 'education that is worthwhile and offers to learners the 'good' of human nourishment'.

> As civilised human beings, we are the inheritors, neither of an inquiry about ourselves and the world, nor of an accumulating body of information, but of a conversation, begun in the primeval forests and extended and made more articulate in the course of centuries. It is a conversation which goes on both in public and within each of ourselves. (Oakeshott, 1959: 197.)

Particularly we espouse two key ideas that guide our thinking about education: that we (amongst many) would define worthwhile education as a practice with impact; and that education should be conducted within the moral mode of practice (Carr, D., 2004).

Worthwhile education as a practice with impact

Endemic to the word 'education' – whenever it is used as precisely as possible — is the notion that the learning involved is intrinsically worthwhile and has positive impact on the learner. Where this is the case, such learning is transformational of the learner (and sometimes for the teacher). It changes and deepens understanding to the point where the learner's conduct — not just surface behaviour —becomes changed. Although that in turn might well make for greater complexity in the learner's conception of what life is about, it nurtures and enriches the learner as a person. It is this that makes teaching a virtuous activity. We indicate carefully how we use 'worthwhile', because modern usage of 'education' seems generally to mean little more than that teacher has transferred information to a passive learner.

We would further argue that a practice cannot be claimed as *educational* unless it is underpinned by (implicit or explicit) understanding of what it is 'to act educationally'. It is broadly agreed that to act educationally is to engage in the deliberate intention to:

- open minds, liberate thinking, encourage critique, explore the foundations of good practice and develop creativity and to nurture and involve the learner in intrinsic motivation (carrot not stick!).

See for example the work of Carr, D. (2003;2004). Carr, W. (1995), Dewey, J. (1897; 1910/1933; 1916), Freire, P. (1970; 1998), Hansen, D. (2001), Oakeshott, M. (1959), Palmer, PJ, (1998), Van Manen, M. (1997; 2015) and Wright, T and Fish, D. (2105).

Thus, where learners are enabled to think in broader rather than narrower terms, have their confidence well-grounded and fuelled rather than drained, and have their engagement with the world deepened — then their teachers may, irrespective of their educational 'know-how' or skills, claim to practise in an educational way. (See Carr, W., 1995: 160.)

This also means that where learners are not so developed, no amount of technically well-performed teaching skills and clever strategies will compensate, and no technical know-how will make the experience educational for learners.

Therefore, to engage in an educational practice is far beyond simply 'knowing how to do educational things' (having the 'skills' of teaching). For example, instruction of learners can be skilfully performed *but it will not be an educational practice at all*, if it has been used to impose a process upon learners who have been required to ignore their personal perspectives including their own values, attitudes and feelings, suspend their thinking, shut down their critical faculties, abandon their moral awareness, and merely parrot a performance.

This would not conform to ethical educational principles of procedure concerned with cultivating the *understanding* which enables learners to explore and come to their own view about why, how, where and when to use that skill, which in turn commits them to develop or change their practice. Indeed, it would be training, not education. Thus, '*training in a particular skill* may or may not be educational, depending on the extent to which it opens up the mind and contributes to that growth as a person' (Pring, 2000).

This is why 'education' is significantly different from 'training'. By the same token, 'conduct' (one's overt way of being in the world, that arises from one's inner beliefs and values) is significantly different from one's 'behaviour' (our visible actions that spring from what an outside agent has told us what and how to do). And in that sense educators cannot avoid (though they might try to ignore) the moral nature of educational practice.

Education in the moral mode of practice

We see teaching as a moral and intellectual practice within a rich tradition that goes back to the Greeks in the centuries before Christ. The argument, with acknowledgements to Hanson (2001) is as follows.

i. To focus only on the *means* of teaching (the 'how to') is sterile. It then becomes: a job with a task to transmit knowledge; an occupation where those outside it set the terms and conditions and the activities to be carried out.

ii. To focus instead only on the ends, can lead to 'outcomes-focused' approaches, where the product is: socialising; acculturating; producing productive members of society, successful and compliant workers. This is dangerous and equally un-educational.

iii. Teaching as a practice has its own integrity — to those who are thoughtful about what they do as teachers.

iv. 'Teachers should first determine what they care about [say the qualities of practising doctors they are 'bringing up'] and then craft a conception of teaching that coheres with that determination.' (Hanson, 2001: 4.)

v. Teachers who give their planning and their practice intellectual and moral substance are also echoing the components of teaching that have developed over time. That is, they are intellectually attentive to learners by focusing on what learners know, can do, feel and think, with an eye to building their knowledge of the world and how to continue to learn within it.

vi. Teachers are morally attentive to learners by being alert to learners' responses to opportunities to *grow as persons* (to become more rather than less thoughtful about ideas, and more rather than less sensitive to others' views and concerns). They are mindful that every learner is unique, with a distinctive set of dispositions, capabilities, understandings and outlooks.

Thus, as Hansen suggests the bonds between teacher and learner are intellectual and moral, pertaining to their emerging knowledge, understanding and growth as persons, and so the concept *'person'* is central to the practice of teaching. Teachers conduct themselves like this, not as a means to an end, but because that is what they see as *'being a teacher'*. (Hansen, 2001.) Biesta has more recently also continued on this theme, (Biesta, 2010).

Teaching in the moral mode of postgraduate medical educational practice

Emerging from these arguments are three key things that are vital for medical educators to aim for.

1. **Making explicit for yourself**, the human and humane as well as the technical aspects of patients' needs; the human and humane as well as the technical demands of medical practice in all its complexity; and therefore identifying the educational imperatives to be working on with learning doctors.

2. **Seeing educational practice as** attending to learners' *being* and *becoming* as persons, and to their thinking and decision making processes, as well as to their learning of knowledge and skills defined in their curriculum; recognising that — in addition, or even opposition, to what you say — *your being as a doctor and a teacher* will have a profound impact on your learner as an important model for that learner; being an advocate for the kind of education necessary for developing a wise doctor (one who practises with the best interests of the whole patient at their heart, using their expertise with sound professional judgement to tailor the care they offer to the patient's own circumstances).

3. **Having clarified for oneself** what does and does not conduce to engaging in education and medicine in the moral mode of practice; being committed to work to support worthwhile PGME and where necessary to resist the narrowness of the demands made by the curriculum, by the pressure of daily practice, by the expectations of the NHS, government, Royal Colleges, and the media; being committed to educating the wise doctor if necessary in opposition to any requirements of external agents that are inimical to this.

In summary, we see *the moral mode of practice in Postgraduate Medical Education* as about aspiring to:

- understand and make explicit for yourself how you see the practice of medicine
- understand what kinds of education will conduce to developing a wise doctor
- critique what external agents (national curricula etc) require and where necessary seeing these as mere basic requirements and seeking to enrich them in ways which ensure that the learner is nurtured in becoming a holistic doctor.

An overview of reflection on practice

This book, building on the ideas of key authors (Dewey, Schön, Proctor, Grundy, Moon, Bolton etc) sees reflection on practice as *the central educational process* through which any professional practitioner can explore and learn, both from and through their own practice. It is not simply a bolt-on adjunct to learning to become a professional practitioner. Reflection means exploring (enquiring in a disciplined way into) examples of our own practice and comparing this with agreed professional ideals, in order to gain meaningful understanding of both that piece of practice and of ourselves as the practitioner within it. By this means, reflection should be transformative of practitioners themselves and of their practice, so that the ultimate beneficiaries of this important process become the patients/clients/learners themselves.

Transformation indicates improvement. The process includes uncovering, appreciating and critiquing carefully the very drivers of our actions, thinking, and decision making. It also involves recognising significant moments or elements of what occurred or was thought, and pinpointing their precise significance for the practitioner as learner.

Reflection is thus the most efficient way of gaining far more from one's own practical experience than the mere memory of the facts of the case. This is true for three reasons:

- there is far more to a clinical event than is visible on its surface

- facts of a case are themselves subjective and their provenance needs to be investigated

- in what has been called the 'white heat' of practice (Fish, 2012a: 52), there is, in the moment, never time to think deeply about what is happening.

Indeed, in the giddy pace of practice much has to be processed speedily. The possibilities and choices are fleetingly registered, the potential of various courses of action flash past, the likely complexities are factored-in fast, and the nuances that lie beneath the surface action are noted, if at all, in nanoseconds. Later, snorkelling beneath the surface of that action after the waves have settled, yields unexpected and sometimes surprising riches and even uncovers motives and reasons for decisions that were barely comprehended at the time but make for wiser justification than could have been expressed *in situ*. Thus, having an experience and understanding its meaning do not occur simultaneously. Reflection makes meaning out of experience, makes the invisible visible, and helps to ensure that the fullest and most appropriate learning has been gained from it.

Unfortunately, within postgraduate medical practice this is not how reflection is generally understood, having been attached to processes like assessment and appraisal, without clear indications of how it is to be enacted, or why.

Defining reflection

There is no one simple definition of reflection that does full justice to its nature. However, we can make some general points, which are likely to hold good in all circumstances. For example, we would want to say that in principle, reflection is certainly not the same as meditation, nor is it a quick chat, or even a fast think about what has happened to us in a practice setting, nor is it a collegiate discussion about policy and practice within a department (which can happen when something has gone wrong). All these have their place in learning to practise, but reflection is the means of enquiring in a disciplined way into one's own practice and one's own conduct within it.

Reflection, then, is about:

- exploring what underlies our various different practice experiences and recognising the person and professional we bring to them on different occasions in different contexts

- seeking to uncover rigorously and understand and articulate the relationship between one's visions, values and beliefs, and one's thought, knowledge and action, in reference to specific examples of one's own practice

- having an exploratory cast of mind that is investigative, disciplined, critical and meticulous

- contextualising one's practice, viewing and investigating it critically, and exploring open-mindedly how it relates to wider understandings of that practice and the practice of one's profession

- understanding our thinking in practice better, and thus being motivated and committed to improving it, and thereby being equipped to go about such improvement

- recognising and critiquing the moral dimensions of our own work and the developing nature of our profession.

Reflective practice is thus regarded generally as a special kind of practice, which involves systematic critical enquiry into one's professional work and one's relationship to it, (Fish, 1998).

Choice of focus for reflection

The choice of topic/event should be made for its likely educational impact in respect of one's own practice (though reflection upon practical examples of habits and rituals has important things to teach us too). In that sense, reflective practice will probably not coincide with talking through an adverse medical incident for medico-legal purposes, and it is unlikely to be the same activity as discussion of an event for the purposes of risk management. However, the ability to present evidence of regular inquiry into one's own practice in order to develop it, would in any discussion of a problematic legal or risk management situation, provide significant empirical proof of one's on-going concern for good practice.

As a key means of unearthing all that lies beneath the visible surface of practice, reflection is about *generating knowledge out of practice*.

As an educational process, it enables learners to consider critically and develop those forces that drive their practice, and it ultimately allows them to demonstrate their development for themselves and their teachers/supervisors and provides evidence for their assessment that is more holistic and detailed than merely quantifying their visible skills.

Given the context of the prevailing conditions of the 21st Century, reflection is at last set to become an indispensable part of medical education. For many years it has come as part of the curriculum for most professions but has been slow to be recognised in medical practice, and has yet to be fully used as enabling meaning to be made out of an experience, so that the learning that emerges from ordinary practice is properly enhanced. Even now in medical practice it still tends to be regarded as a means of determining why something went wrong, and the old superficial process of asking "what went well and what went badly?" blinds doctors to the real use and value of properly disciplined reflective processes.

In most professional preparation courses, reflection has been used to balance the training element (which develops pure skills) by attending to the thinking and knowing that needs to underlie them in real clinical activities if the practice is to be truly and consciously intelligent. That is why reflection has been taken up as significant by so many professions. The literature of teaching, nursing, occupational therapy, physiotherapy and a wide range of other professions related to medicine, has long been full of serious contributions to this field. Medical Education, particularly at postgraduate level, now not only needs to catch up but to make its own unique contribution. This is because, as this book shows, reflection on medical practice needs to acknowledge the unique role of the doctor in decision making. It therefore requires processes that focus in more detail on key professional judgements and what underpins these. However, this is not to say that the processes outlined in this book, might not be of considerable use to all kinds of professional practitioners (Fish and Boniface, 2012).

Reflection on practice then, is a means of enabling practitioners to:

- explore, make sense of, and thus understand more fully their current experiences, actions and events

- contextualise these current experiences and relate them critically to other relevant theory and practice
- extend their current competence in clinical practice
- recognise new challenges to work on in clinical practice
- appreciate the subtleties of clinical practice
- connect particular practice experiences, events and activities to wider ideas and ideals of practice across their profession
- develop a personal vision of clinical practice
- provide evidence of growing insight and progress in understanding
- crystallise and summarise progress at the end of various stages of learning.

But all this occurs only under certain conditions, and only when the purpose of reflection is itself educational, as opposed to concerned with health care management or therapeutic relief (see Proctor, 1986).

As they learn their practice, doctors daily engage in, or are party to, a wide range of activities in the clinical setting. These include: having a particular experience, being involved in an event, carrying out an action, learning or practising a skill or skills. But their practice is holistic. These things all happen together, happen fast and fluently, and many of the elements involved are invisible, and so undergoing these activities, is not the same as understanding them. Indeed, it would be possible to go through many of them, without engaging the mind at all, rather as we sometimes find when we have driven somewhere on auto-pilot not consciously noticing the detail of the route because our mind has been elsewhere.

It is possible to have the experience but to fail to make meaning out of it by failing to:

- notice the finer points of it
- recognise the principles that can be drawn from it
- make links between it and other relevant occurrences or previous learning
- see or sort out and consider the salient elements in it.

Considerably more value will be extracted from clinical practice, where reflection enables the learner to focus intelligently upon it in order to make meaning out of it (understand it). In the early stages of a practitioner's career, this reflection needs to be shared and validated by reference to the experience of more senior practitioners. It should be remembered that new learners do not always make the same profound sense out of something that experts have long seen as having significant features. Indeed, while one part of education is about encouraging learners to recognise and share their visions of their current achievements, another part is about enabling them to see more and differently than they would if left alone, and to help them tease out meanings and significances that they would otherwise miss.

There are other reasons too for engaging in reflection as part of learning in clinical settings. As members of a profession, doctors work with and for vulnerable people (patients). This brings special responsibilities. For the sake of their patients, therefore, they need to:

- be able to dig their theories and values out from under their practice, in order to examine, explore and even challenge them
- recognise when their practice doesn't match up to their theories and values
- be a seeker rather than a knower
- recognise their uncertainties and use them as growing-points
- step back and take a long view of themselves and their practice
- explore the qualities of professionalism and consider how they match up to their own.

All this includes looking at the kind of person one is: one's virtues, dispositions, habits of mind, shortcomings, capacities, values, beliefs, theories, ideas, attitudes, commitments, ideals, principles, feelings, understandings, imagination and criticality.

Reflection and the moral implications of practice

Reflection inevitably involves standing back from our practice — *and ourselves as part of that practice* — and exploring and challenging both that practice and our beliefs, assumptions, expectations, feelings, attitudes and values as they impact on our practice. Such reflection examines not merely the facts of the case but our thinking and decision making within it, as well as our very being as a practitioner. Thus, it cannot avoid opening up questions about whether or not our actions were/are morally informed and to what extent they are shaped by a critical consideration of ends and means.

For example, given the current climate, a particularly useful focus for individual medical and surgical practitioners might be determining, within their own practice, which actions are properly and appropriately rule-governed (protocol and guideline led), and which are not. Serious practical enquiry into their own work would equip them with the ability (when needed on the spot):

i. to articulate the arguments for maintaining control over their clinical thought and action (which is always at risk from risk management, quality control and political correctness)

ii. to share powerful and persuasive evidence of the importance of their deliberative and discretionary decisions and their wise judgements.

Reflection also means standing outside the practice of one's profession as a whole and its traditions, and seeing it anew. Grundy (1987) makes this point well when she says that there is a tendency in those who engage in reflection on their actions in a piece of practice:

> to be guided in judgements about that action by an interpretation of the meaning

of the situation which is constrained by traditional meanings....The problem is to act in ways that are not already pre-determined by habitual practice.

Going on to quote Arendt's work she adds:

Action which proceeds from judgement-making is a more authentic form of human endeavour than rule-generating or rule-following behaviour, (Grundy, 1987: 175).

It should be noted however, that we are not saying that reflection is something that can be carried out in depth on all one's practice activities, all the time. More value is likely to emerge from homing in upon a few incidents a month than will come from working in less depth on a greater number. It is, however, worth adopting a mind-set which is always alert to finding a suitable aspect of practice to enquire into.

Various means of engaging in reflection

There are many formats or models and guidelines that offer ways of shaping attempts at reflection, but, as other professions have already found, they are only useful in the early stages while practitioners find their own voice.

In general, the key modes of engaging in reflection are talking and writing. Reflection is essentially dialogic and thrives on interaction. It develops through being shared and being worked over and refined. That is why talking something through reflectively will help, and why written dialogue through e-mails is beginning to support postgraduate medical learners in their early practice.

A record of such reflective dialogue cannot be recalled or refined at a later date. The detail and nuance of the talking will be lost. We argue therefore that there is no substitute for producing and refining an extended piece of writing from time to time, because it reveals more as you go along, and anyone can do it. The most difficult thing is starting; once professionals have begun this process, they rarely abandon it.

Table 1.2.1 offers a range of characteristics which are typical of authentic engagement in reflective practice.

Table 1.2.1 Some defining characteristics of reflective practice
(Adapted and extended from Moon, 1999: 64-65)

- The subject matter should be one's own practice and its particular context.
- Reflection involves investigating practice systematically and critically from as many points of view as possible (re-viewing it).
- It involves standing back from practice and offers the possibility of thinking about it from outside the existing traditions or established patterns of practice.
- It is about practitioners coming to an understanding of their actions, their espoused theories and theories-in-use.
- It includes moral questions about the worthwhile nature of activities themselves, and thus attends to ends as well as means.
- Reflection should always consider the person and professional that the practitioner brings to this particular event.
- Reflection should not generalise across several events or days of practice, rather it is specific to a given event and context.
- Like a case in case-study research, it should be clearly 'bounded', so that the case/event/clinical experience being reflected upon should have a clear beginning and an end (even if it is an event within a longer patient pathway).
- Reflection is likely to be triggered by uncertainty about something in the mind of the practitioner.
- It will engage with moral and ethical content (professional work being morally centred).
- It will be precipitated by questions/tasks/personal considerations/problematic issues, to which there is no simple solution.
- It will engage in critique of practice.
- Its intention is the attainment of better understanding in the context of improving practice generally.
- It is not just about thinking, but articulating that thinking in spoken or written form and as a result, being able to extend, refine and develop it.
- It is enhanced when shared with others.

Successful reflection demands all of the following: description, analysis, interpretation, appreciation, self-awareness, self-criticism, imagination, creativity and synthesis.

Reflection for doctors

Reflection on personal professional practice as a central core in learning to practice and to develop it, is key to ensuring that we give patients the best possible service we can. In what way then is reflection a different process for you as a doctor compared with other healthcare professionals? And what can it do for you?

Reflection for medical practice

It is important that doctors do not automatically take as models for their own reflective processes, the work and ideas of other healthcare professions. The design of reflection for medical practice requires a recognition that both the role of the doctor and the specific nature of medical practice are unique.

The nature of medical practice has at its heart:

- ultimate responsibility for the individual patient's medical treatment and care

- the exercise of discretion in key and often crucial professional judgements about patient care

- ultimate professional decision making about diagnosis and treatment

- final responsibility for the whole care of the patient

- a litigious and media climate that places doctors as first in line of responsibility for the health of the nation.

Unlike all other healthcare professionals, who once qualified and registered for a full career, immediately beginning continuing professional development, doctors first undergo a long undergraduate period followed by as many as twelve or more years in postgraduate practice. Here they follow formal specialty curricula and are thus under professional education and assessment processes. Throughout this postgraduate practice, reflection should be a central means of learning to grow as a doctor. Only after this, as consultants, can they engage in continuing professional development, which should also include reflection on practice as a means of becoming a better practitioner.

Reflection in healthcare more generally

Reflective Practice in healthcare professions other than medicine is much more well-developed and researched. We summarise our comments about them, based on considerable experience of working with other health practitioners and making contributions to their developing practices (Benner, 1984; Driscoll, 2000; Epstein, 1999; Fish, 2012b; Fish and Twinn, 1997; Higgs, 1990; 2003; Higgs and Jones, 2002; Higgs, Fish and Rothwell, 2004; 2007; Johns, 1995; Mattingly and Fleming, 1994; Rolfe and Freshwater, 2001; Ryan, 1995).

- Reflection as produced by healthcare practitioners tends to offer a relatively uncritical narrative, focused on an overview of their practice.

- It mainly sets out to tell the story or offer a description of an event, or a morning, or an incident — as seen from the reflector's point of view, and chronicled after the event either orally or in writing.

- It may or may not have a critical edge and often does not pinpoint the crucial elements of an event, and is often so caught up in 'applying' professional theory automatically to their practice that the wider, and sometimes more human picture, is lost.

- Its structure is usually chronological, must be autobiographical and its style should be narrative-descriptive.

- Its purpose is to report on what has happened, how the reflector has responded to this, and to think about it more carefully (and perhaps to do it differently next time).

- In written form it records events (actions, activities, occurrences) within the writer's experience, but it does not usually focus in great detail on their underlying drivers.

Reflection of this kind has been unfairly seen by doctors as a 'fluffy' activity, engaged in mainly by non-medical staff. At its best it can be useful, but is not often very deep.

Reflection as useful for medical practice

Medical practice requires doctors to be wise professionals who engage in complex thinking, make wise, far-reaching and crucial decisions and come to often irreversible professional judgements about what to do with (or where necessary even on behalf of) their patients.

This means that as a doctor, you are relied upon to:

- understand and take careful account of the values that drive your practice

- understand the importance of context because everything is context specific and your interpretation of happenings and comments is based on your (often subconscious) formulation of the underlying agenda, made at an early stage on quite flimsy evidence

- articulate the thinking that underpins your decision making, which may well go far beyond following protocols

- make your own wise professional judgements, not just do what someone else wants (even sometimes when it is the patient who 'wants')

- thus, recognise the crucial difference between patients' 'wants' and 'needs'

- create a therapeutic relationship with each patient, which goes beyond safe patient care, to caring about that individual patient

- have considerable self-knowledge not just be skilled and medically knowledgeable

- recognise the moral dimensions of your practice and strive for *praxis*, where you are relied upon to be 'a good person' who 'does your work well' for its own sake and not for reward.

In summary then, in order to support a doctor's striving towards this set of ideals, the reflective processes that doctors engage in must be focused on these matters. This crucially requires the demonstration of considerable self-awareness and character, as well as the ability to unpack the complex thinking, decisions and judgements that are made in a given situation, and to reconsider them where necessary. That is why reflection for doctors is so different. It enables you to:

- dig your theories and values out from under your practice, in order to examine, explore and even challenge them (or to recognise that your practice doesn't match up to your theories and values)

- uncover rigorously and understand and articulate the relationship between your visions, values and beliefs, and your thought, knowledge and action, in reference to specific examples of your own practice

- recognise your uncertainties and use them as growing-points

- explore the qualities of professionalism and consider yourself against them

- look at the kind of person you are: your virtues, dispositions, habits of mind, shortcomings, capacities, values, beliefs, theories, ideas, attitudes, commitments, ideals, principles, feelings, understandings, imagination and criticality

- develop and be able to articulate your own personal vision of clinical practice.

Endnote

It will already be apparent that systematic and rigorous reflection on professional practice has a considerable history. The next chapter looks briefly at the key educational thinkers associated with it, showing how their ideas have developed, and also offers a glimpse into the history of some professions, showing how reflective practice has established itself as a valuable process in practice development (albeit one which itself is properly open to critical scrutiny and comes with costs as well as benefits). It is not offered in the expectation that readers will pursue these authors, but rather that they recognise the width and depth of serious writing about reflection, and its provenance.

Chapter Three

Historical Perspectives: the development of ideas about reflection as a practice

Introduction
Key thinkers in the development of reflection on practice
The changing focus of reflection
Endnote

Introduction

This chapter provides an overview of the development of reflection on practice and is offered in two sections. Please note that an overview of ideas is *not the same as a literature review*! It should be noted that any overview of historical trends in any subject is inevitably shaped by the individual writers' own experiences, values and interests. That is, it is interpretive, being coloured by the authors' perceptions of and ways of identifying and categorising, key writers and events.

The first section sets out a critical historical review of the development of ideas about reflection from the Greek philosophers through to modern times, and ends with a focus on reflection within healthcare and medical practice. The second section offers a view of the changing focus of reflection as a practice, identifying four stages in the modern development of reflection. It seems to us that many medical educators do not have a clear understanding of such details as offered below.

We should also mention, and will pick up in more detail later (see Section Three, Chapter Nine), that during much of the last 30 years and in patches even before that, many professionals were taught a seriously flawed notion of what education is about, which has had deleterious effects. Thus, currently not only the youngest doctors schooled in the UK or under UK systems but even those in mid-career are 'products' of a society, shaped by the ideas embedded in the construction and implementation of school/assessment systems (and, to an increasing level, likewise its university systems). These do not promote the 'nurturing' of the humane, independent thinker, but rather promote a reliance on authority. We will need to remember that such doctors would perhaps feel rudderless if not told what to do, and have probably looked (without success) to be told in this way about reflective practice.

What we offer here therefore is our interpretation of the development of ideas about reflection, designed to enable readers to see the context in which this book has come to life. We are *not* recommending that what follows should become 'knowledge transferred' to current doctors. But we should remember that some more enterprising doctors may have met one or two of the approaches to reflection offered below and treated them as 'the' way forward.

Key thinkers in the development of reflection on practice

The concept of learning through experience goes back to the Greeks and was significantly shaped by Aristotle's ideas of *praxis*. This is practical activity directed ultimately towards the achievement of a virtue (a good in society, like an educated person), rather than following a protocol towards the making or building of something preconceived in detail, like a boat or a house. *Praxis* therefore is a form of doing that is created *as it progresses in situ*, drawing on appropriate expertise to respond to individual growth. It is inevitably morally informed, morally committed action. Its ends are progressively revised as the 'goods' intrinsic to practice endlessly develop. Such ends are therefore determinable beforehand only in principle. However, in this kind of practical action, what shapes the expertise brought to this kind of practical activity and makes it intelligible to others, is *tradition* — 'the inherited and largely unarticulated body of practical knowledge which constitutes the traditions within which the good intrinsic to that practice is enshrined'. Carr adds:

> [to] practise .... is always a matter of being initiated into the knowledge, understandings and beliefs bequeathed by that tradition through which the practice has been conveyed to us in its present shape.' (Carr, W., 1995: 68.)

But to practise is not only to 'act within a tradition'! It is also to critique that tradition and contribute to its evolution. Indeed, it is the very continuing presence of contesting philosophical viewpoints that provides the oppositional tension, which is essential for critical thinking. To critique something is firstly to recognise carefully and chart the detail of how it works, secondly it is to bring to this a range of ways of analysing and interpreting it in order to appreciate it as fully as possible, and thirdly it is to critique it by considering both how it fits its present tradition and how it might be seen and used to the betterment of practice within and beyond that tradition. Reflecting on experience is itself a practice, which is why the process is referred to as 'Reflective Practice'. It has its own traditions but also critiques these in the light of new understandings and thus it is a developing tradition — just as is the practice of medicine, or of teaching or of law. That is why it is important to understand the development of reflective means and ends.

Further, in a professional context like medical practice, reflection is not simply about learning from one's practice and improving that practice. It is also one means of preventing one's profession from being reduced to accepting as unopposed, a list of elements of practice and an account of what to do and how to do it, constructed by those who are largely outside the profession's current practice but who purport to have resolved all tensions about what characterises medical work in order to render it unproblematic and thus to control it.

For a different and more general view of reflection as a practice, readers are referred to Bolton and Delderfield (2018) which, being the fourth edition of this work, offers a refined and up-to-date handbook that focuses on reflection for professional development generally and the role of writing in particular.

Key thinkers about reflection on practice

Please note that although there has been much written in recent years by many people, particularly about the role of reflection in a wide range of current professional practices, this overview is focused on the key thinkers about reflection on their own practice, who have, in our view, shaped reflection for their time and thus moved that thinking on.

The ideas of Aristotle about *praxis* have more recently been elaborated and developed over more than a century in the work particularly of Dewey, 1897;1910;1916; Habermas, 1971;1972;1974; Kolb, 1984; Gibbs, 1988; Boud, Keogh and Walker, 1985; Van Manen, 1977; 2015; and Schön, 1983;1987;1991. The following offers a brief glimpse of their contributions. All of them are within the broad tradition that holds it important that people become personally engaged in the learning process and that this broadly involves: 're-viewing' a piece of one's own practical experience, thinking about it anew and in some way improving future practice.

Dewey and Habermas

The work of Dewey (1859-1952) has been described as 'the backbone of the study of reflection' (Moon, 1999:11), and he is generally regarded as the father of modern reflective practice. It is interesting to note that all the ideas fundamental to reflective practice come to us through John Dewey who was an American psychologist, philosopher and educator. By contrast, Jurgen Habermas (whose main relevant writings appeared in the early 1970s), was a European sociologist and philosopher. Since Aristotle would have claimed to be working in these whole areas of thought, there being no such divisions in his day, we can thus claim that the founding influences of modern reflective practice are philosophy, psychology and sociology.

Both men were interested in how reflection generates knowledge, but they described reflection in different ways and were interested in it for different reasons. Dewey's work focused on the processes of reflection, and saw its motivation as coming from perplexity about practice, in order to make sense of the world. For him, reflection was an active, persistent and careful consideration of belief and knowledge. His writing on reflection uses metaphors of creation, construction, or reconstruction of new identities and meanings, rather than mirror metaphors of re-presentation, image formation, or copying what already exists. He emphasised the link between thought (as reflection) and action in the development of practice. His ideas were essentially about educational development, where reflection was a natural part of basic educational processes. He saw reflection as a form of problem-solving, (asking questions about practice, theorising it and testing out the theories in an open-minded way). Dewey's key educational books include: *My Pedagogic Creed* (1897); *How We Think* (1910; revised ed., 1933); and *Democracy and Education* (1916), of which the second listed is most centrally on reflection.

For Habermas, reflection was a tool to be used in developing particular forms of knowledge. His work drives towards the ideals of the empowerment and emancipation of the practitioner. For him, reflection is about critique, evaluation and liberation. His key work in this field is to be found in his: *Towards a Rational Society* (1971); *Knowledge and Human Interests* (1972); and *Theory and Practice* (1974). He sees knowledge not as out there waiting to be found but as something which people construct together.

Kolb and Gibbs

Dewey's work gave rise to Kolb's famous ideas about a 'reflective cycle' (an early model of reflection), which carries a rather simplistic view that reflection is generated by experience and that this, once recognised, feeds back into developed practice and then back into reflection. The key points on his cycle (which were represented round a circle) were: concrete experience; reflective observation; abstract conceptualisation; and active experimentation (Kolb, 1984). Kolb's work was specifically developed within the field of experiential education (where the focus is on learning through activities), and was taken up within the education of professionals, where a practice was being learnt or developed. He was concerned not so much with the details of practice, as creating a simple narrative (a description of what had happened), analysing that for the good and bad aspects of it, resolving to improve and learn from this, and thus changing the next practice. This carries within it the notion of 'the simple application of theory to practice', but this does not work in professional practice because no event is ever the same twice.

Kolb's ideas were extended by Gibbs in 1988, to include the following points in a continuous cycle or spiral: description (what happened?); feelings; evaluation (what was good or bad about the experience?); analysis; conclusion (what else would you have done?); and action plan (if it arose again, what would you do?). This cycle adds more detail to Kolb's work. It explores experience in terms of feelings as well as action but still implies that it is possible to apply directly and quickly to practice that which has been learnt, thus still assuming an applicatory relationship between theory and practice, (an idea that we, as authors, reject within the context of learning to be a practitioner).

Boud, Keogh & Walker and Van Manen

Other work which was founded on Dewey's ideas and which cannot be ignored even in the briefest summary, is that of, and Boud, Keogh and Walker in the 1980s and Van Manen in the 1990s and on. In Boud, Keogh and Walker (1985), for the first time, reflection is specifically seen as turning experience into learning both for individuals learning a professional practice and those already practising. This work shows that professionals can improve their *praxis* by scrutinising as much as possible one specific event from their everyday practice. This is the first modern example of reflection in the context of *praxis* and with a real educational intention rather than a concern to learn or improve skills. Their useful book offers a wide range of examples of this, and indicates the costs in terms and resources, as well as the benefits of Reflective Practice.

Van Manen's work offered a reflective model of a different shape from those of Kolb and Gibbs, and with an ethical concern built into it. He saw reflection as hierarchical rather than circular, and contributes the notion of levels of reflection: the first level is about practical concerns in terms of what works; the second is concerned with evaluation of action and belief (practice and theory) and the debating of principles and goals; the third is concerned with ethical and political matters (the link between practice and broader social issues); and (later) the fourth is concerned with meta-level understanding (higher level ideas about thinking). He broadly characterised reflection as mindfulness or attentiveness to practice, and continues to offer perspectives on the phenomenology of practice. (Van Manen, 2014; 2015).

Equally importantly, Van Manen (1992) also helped us to see the importance of narrative as the basis of enquiry into practice and therefore as related to reflection. He thus explicitly linked reflection and the individual practitioner. As Moon (2018:78) neatly says: 'Narrative is an account which describes or explains a [personal] event, narrated afterwards, bringing together different elements, making a whole, and therefore sense out of them'. She also importantly makes a distinction between an incident and an event.

We would say that where an incident is a very short encounter that can be seen out of context, an event has a beginning, a middle and an end and can only be appreciated in context. It is in re-viewing the event, to turn it into a narrative that enables us to reconstruct it with greater sharpness. For example, in recounting and struggling to chart accurately the chronology of an event, we notice and capture small elements as for the first time, and see meaning in the tone of voice and its nuances and become aware of the significance of certain actions and the order of them. Powerful examples of this can be found particularly in the writers of reflection on healthcare. See the work of Hunter, Charon, Frank and Clandinen and Connelly.

The work of Schön

Donald Schön, is probably the most influential thinker on reflection in the last five decades and could be seen as the father of Reflective Practice across all professions. He too recognised the importance of narrative in the process of reflection. His key books are: *The Reflective Practitioner* (1983); *Educating the Reflective Practitioner* (1987), which outlined his main thinking; and *The Reflective Turn* (1991), which provides case studies in and on educational practice. He particularly focused on the preparation of professionals for a career in practice and particularly on their learning in, and from, the practice setting. He specifically explored with them and guided how thy thought while acting (which he called 'reflection-in-action'). Because his work with learners was in real practice and was carried out as a professional conversation, his focus was only concerned with oral reflection.

Professional practice he characterised as the 'swampy lowlands' because practice happens in the indeterminate zone (of life), and is always by definition, complex and incomplete. This in itself was a concept, well characterised by its label, that enabled some practitioners for the first time to acknowledge that being an expert was not about being certain, but was rather about the inevitability that not all can ever be known about individual human beings and the complexity of their lives and their professional practices. This of course is particularly significant in medical and healthcare practice. Thus, Schön highlighted a more down-to-earth understanding of the nature of professional practice, and therefore saw the importance of context in considering and learning from practical experience.

Schön's work, though much critiqued, has contributed most to the general drive to incorporate reflection into the teaching of professional practice in professional settings. He has teased apart the artistry from the rule-following 'craft or rationality' of practice, which he saw as dangerous. From him we get the idea of reflection-in-action (the thinking that happens when actions do not go according to plan) and reflection-on-action (reflection that occurs after the action), and the need for professionals to learn in a 'sheltered practicum' (an experience of practice where the student has a taste of real practice but does not bear the full responsibility for every aspect of the work). Schön described the main features of a practicum as: 'learning by doing, coaching rather than teaching, and a dialogue of reciprocal reflection-in-action between coach and student' (Schön, 1987, p 303).

Schön's work has been criticised for using imprecise terms (there is debate about what reflection-in-action really means, and his definition seems too narrow), and on the grounds that his practical examples do not exactly match his theorising. For example, Eraut, (1995), wishes to reject the term 'reflection' as Schön uses it, and Greenwood, (1993), points out inconsistencies (in his work with Argyris) between Schön's ideas and his actual pedagogical interventions as described and recommended in his work. Interestingly, Greenwood recommends that nurse educators should follow Schön's theorising rather than his practice. Nonetheless, Schön's work was pioneering, and remains seminal for those who educate professionals in the practice setting.

Some key writers on reflective practice in healthcare and medicine

In the last two decades of the twentieth century in the Western world, the work of Schön, and these earlier key thinkers became gradually recognised and more and more influential on those in professional practice in healthcare, who use reflection for a wide variety of purposes. That is probably why in the first two decades of our current century, influential books on reflection *as a practice* have given way to thousands of journal articles and conference papers all reporting on the use of reflection in professional practice settings, and what has been learnt from it and about it. This writing is mainly at the micro level and tends to argue for or commend protocols and guidelines for specific use in particular professional practice settings. It also explores inter-professional practice settings to discuss the practical problems in trying to assess reflection in specific contexts.

One further trend however, does need to be noted — that of the linking of reflection to enquiry into professional practice. This sees reflection as a process that is valuable for some forms of qualitative research. Some in this field claim that reflection is itself a *form* of qualitative research, but we do not find this a persuasive argument because it seems to rule out the significance and use of multiple perspectives, which we would see as one essential key principle of good humanistic enquiry.

The history of the development of reflection in healthcare, although it goes back at least 35 years in Britain, America and Australia, has not yet been fully charted. The following are recognised as key writers on reflection for undergraduate practice placements: Benner, (1984); Carper, (1978); Driscoll, (2000); Fish and Twinn, 1997; Fish, Twinn and Purr, (1990); Johns, (1995); Rolfe and Freshwater (2001) in nursing; Higgs (who has published a wide range of books in the 1990s and early 21st Century in physiotherapy and healthcare generally); Mattingly and Fleming, (1994), Ryan (1995), Bonniface and Seymour, (2012) in occupational therapy.

Some of this work still relies heavily on Kolb and Gibbs rather than later thinkers, and this is still given motivation and emphasis within the design of many curriculums of undergraduate professional preparation degrees, where writing about practice is required and undergraduates still seem to be seen as needing very simplistic frameworks. However, many of these authors have also been involved in developing postgraduate work in the practice setting as 'Professional development' and at profession-specific masters level courses where a number of PhDs from across these professions are based on a reflective methodology and are available now on the shelves of a number of university libraries or on digital record.

Reflection for postgraduate practitioners includes the work of Karen Mann and Della Freeth on inter-professional working, as well as Fish and Coles (1998). Fish and Coles offer a range of case studies on professional judgement in a range of individual professions, all of which reflect on professional judgement in practice.

Postgraduate medicine by comparison with all these, has been (apart from Law) the slowest profession to embrace reflection as having a major role in learning. There are so far, only a handful of names to report across the entire medical field, and all their work is very recent. The key figures on reflection in medical education are: (from America) Epstein's 1999 work on 'mindful practice', which is an excellent summary of how reflective practice relates to medicine; (from Australia) the work of Cox, (1999), in surgery; (from Britain) the work of Downey and Macnaughton, eds (2001); and in medicine generally Greenhalgh and Hurwitz, eds (1998); West, (2001) and Launer, (2015) offer work on reflection in general practice; and White and Stancombe (2003), in paediatrics. In addition, it should be recognised that the writing of Gawande, (2001), in surgery (produced in America but published in Britain) is also in the reflective tradition, although he does not make this explicit. The work of Fish and de Cossart, (2005, 2007,

2011 (eds), 2012, 2013) on developing reflection for teachers in postgraduate medical practice is discussed in the next chapter.

These writers are read mainly by those on masters courses in education in clinical settings for medical consultants and other senior medical staff, in which reflective practice is an integral component. More and more PhDs are appearing in the field of medical education on the artistry of practice. The value of Reflective Practice to postgraduate medicine has yet to be truly appreciated and respected.

The changing focus of reflection: four developmental stages

This part of the chapter firstly considers briefly the traditions of reflective practice which seem to emerge from the above overview, and shows the key stages of the development of reflection as a practice (though they were not separated stages but overlapping ones). Secondly it considers the gradual sharpening of focus about the intentions for reflecting on practice. Finally, and taking account of the above overview, it offers examples of three different styles of written reflection that are contingent upon those differing intentions.

The developing traditions of reflective practice seem to us to fall into four sections, each of which has its own protagonists who drew attention to specific characteristics of reflection as a practice, each enriching our understanding of the ideas. We explore this under four headings:

- the Foundation stage: reflection as a form of thinking and knowing
- the structural and technical stage: reflection by mantra
- the narrative and descriptive stage: story-telling without the full power of narrative
- the educationally transformative stage.

The Foundation stage: reflection as a form of thinking and knowing

Clearly, one does not read the work of either Dewey or of Habermas to 'learn how to do reflection'. These writers are foundational at a theoretical level, which, though essential to a thorough understanding of the whole development of the field of Reflective Practice, are not central to the practice of reflection except as the originators of ideas waiting to be linked to educational intentions.

Dewey's writing offers a philosophical basis for reflection by elaborating the philosophical principles of 'good education'. He sees reflection as a *form* of thinking. He claims that the elements of Reflective Thinking are: "a) a state of perplexity, hesitation, doubt: and b) an act of search or investigation directed towards bringing to light further facts which serve to corroborate or to nullify the suggested belief" (Dewey, 1910: 9). He adds 'Demand for the solution of a perplexity is the steadying and guiding factor in the entire process of reflection' (Dewey, 1910: 11). He explores the place of thinking in experience here and also in *Democracy and Education* (1916), but these explorations are at a deeply philosophical level, and do not discuss practice. The same is true of Habermas, whose main contributions were in the traditions of critical theory and pragmatism.

The structural and technical stage: reflection by mantra

It was Kolb and Gibbs who created a practical way forward. In response to the ideas of Dewey, Kolb sought to link experience *as if observed in real practice*, to an evaluation of that experience, in order to create an improved approach to the next experience. Here the narrative that offers a true story of an event in practice is seen as the important issue. Further, Kolb's very simple early version of the reflective cycle contained at least three flaws: it overlooked the significance of the invisible elements of an event (like the thinking and decision making involved); it assumed that the scope of an experience could be done full justice to by reporting the key visible facts (which of course leaves out much of the human side of the experience); it saw learning from one experience as directly applied to the next (which misunderstands the complexity of experience itself and ignores the facts that no two experiences are ever exactly the same). This is why Gibbs' reflective cycle, though still very simplistic, was somewhat better in that it recognised the importance of the practitioner's feelings (though not their thoughts!). However, this rather heavily guided approach did give rise to both oral and written modes of reflection, because it could be created relatively easily in either mode.

The narrative and descriptive stage: story-telling without the full power of narrative

The influence of Kolb and Gibbs has been responsible between about 1980 and 2010 for many healthcare practitioners taking a narrative and descriptive approach to reflection which has in some cases been somewhat superficial. Capturing the facts of the event/case were often the single motive for engaging in reflection. Reflection here was simply something required as a slightly puzzling part of learning that would somehow improve their behaviour in the next practice event. The idea seemed to be to capture the story of an aspect of or a period of time in their own practice and to tell it as vividly and descriptively as possible. There was often little guidance of what to include in this or what to do with it afterwards, and it easily degenerated to the somewhat boring reporting of a series of incidents — particularly, as often happened, when the narrative itself was seen as the end product, and not explored in any way. However, the enjoyment of story-telling did encourage greater enjoyment of the reflective writing process.

The outcome of this was that reflection gained a poor reputation in postgraduate medical education and was seen as 'soft and fuzzy' when first introduced. Doctors also balked at the idea of spending time writing something in which they saw no value because the worthwhile educational intentions of the process had not been explained to them.

The best work in this field however, comes from: Charron (2006); Clandinin and Connelly (2000); Frank (1995); Hunter (1993) and Montgomery, (2006). In these cases an enriched narrative is the basis of their work. Our Transformative Reflection lies, to some extent, within this tradition.

The educationally transformative stage

All the previous three stages as well as the work of Boud, Keogh and Walker and particularly Schön, have contributed to the drive to create a much more valuable and properly rigorous approach to Reflective Practice. They have also lent significance to the recognition that the purpose for reflection needs to be clear, the style of writing required by it needs to be understood, and the tailoring of it to the specific educational needs of different professions needs to be thought through and made explicit. Its moral dimensions also need to be recognised and considered.

In other words, it needs to attend to the depth of thought and the complexity and uncertainty as well as the moral dilemmas that are part of any professional practice that serves human beings and strives for their good. This is why real education is transformative. It develops the whole person whom the practitioner brings to their work. We refer to this as changing the learner's conduct (action driven by personal beliefs and values), rather than altering their behaviour (which may be the result of outside pressure and will only be permanent if it truly reflects their own choice and thus becomes conduct).

Properly rigorous reflection is indispensable in learning to practise — in learning the principles of professional practice itself, in learning about oneself as a practitioner; and in grasping the practical procedures that are part of all professional practice and in seeing practice as a whole. It is also a user-friendly means of exploring one's own achievements, and struggles in coping with the uncertainty and complexity of serving one's patients, learners or clients. It is not about finding fault and assigning blame, but rather about presenting one's experience of everyday events and exploring the expertise shown in them and one's developing insight about how to improve it in medicine. It is about learning to think like a doctor, to recognise who one is as a doctor, to see patients and colleagues as human beings and to conduct oneself accordingly. Such reflection then, needs to begin with a very clear understanding of the educational intentions for engaging in it.

Teacher educators needed only the work of Boud, Keogh and Walker (1985) and of Schön (1987) to make the link with the educational ideas of Dewey, which many teachers already regarded as a key basis of their work. They had quickly seen that reflection on an experience enabled the meaning of it to emerge within the learner. They knew that much-repeated experience which was not explored in detail provided nothing but repetition — and that it could even reinforce error if not properly monitored!

Endnote

This chapter has provided the landscape in which to locate where the ideas offered in this book can be found. What follows introduces our ideas and resources, specifically designed for doctors.

Chapter Four

The Transformative Reflective Process revealed: a detailed introduction

> Introduction
> What TRP offers to doctors that previous reflective processes have failed to provide
> The Principles and Components of TRP
> Transformative Reflection: how the components interrelate
> Our educational thinking now underpinning Transformative Reflection
> The Narrative and Exploratory Invisibles
> A short comment about each of our eight Invisibles
> Endnote

Introduction

The intentions of this chapter are to enable readers both to locate our Transformative Reflective Process (TRP) for doctors and surgeons within the broader landscape of Reflective Practice for the professions, as offered earlier in Part One, and to recognise how its principles are aligned with the processes described there. It also seeks to indicate how we have reconceptualised our own understanding of reflection for doctors in order to ensure that it facilitates their detailed exploration of their practice in a specific case, and therefore how the doctor's expertise can be recognised, appreciated, and critiqued, so as to improve their professional practice in serving patients.

This chapter therefore provides an overview of the principles, components and processes which have led to our reconceived TRP as a particular version of reflective practice for doctors. This prepares readers to engage with them in detail as guided in Part Two.

We acknowledge that these ideas we have developed over many years only represent the Invisibles we have uncovered so far, (de Cossart & Fish, 2005, Fish & de Cossart, 2007, 2013). Being a problematic concept, there may be other ways of seeing this and other Invisibles lurking elsewhere in medical practice (see for example Chapter Twelve). This might even become in itself a new avenue for research.

What TRP offers to doctors that previous reflective processes have failed to provide

Transformative Reflection for doctors is designed to focus doctors' attention on their response to what medical and surgical practice daily demands of them and how this relates to society's ideal aspirations about the consummate professionalism and wisdom of a doctor (see Chapter One). This form of reflection also equips doctors to articulate their own level of expertise within a given case, both for themselves (to aid their own development) and for a range of audiences (to provide them, as appropriate, with a more accurate understanding of the quality of their work and its context, and thus fuel a more reasonable set of expectations of them).

Until now, the medical profession has, as shown in Chapters Two and Three, had little appreciation of what reflection can really do for doctors. This is mainly because the principles, components and processes of earlier forms of reflection, having been borrowed from other professions, have neither contributed well to the education of doctors, nor helped society understand the realities and demands of everyday medical practice. Indeed, mostly until now, reflection used at postgraduate medical education level can be described as:

- attending only to the visible surface of a doctor's practice, ignoring as tacit, its complexity
- useful mainly for formal assessment purposes only
- mainly oral within a supervised session and then summarised in writing to be put on record
- to be done as quickly as possible and without due recognition of its educational and communicative importance and of the time necessary to turn it from a superficial learning experience, (where little is actually learnt), to an in-depth exploration—and therefore development —of the learner's practice in all its complexity
- focused mainly on the learner's understanding of the medical facts and procedures of the case, with little attention to the humanity of either the patient or the doctor
- without deeper critique beyond the discussion of the learner's medical knowledge
- with no recognition of the significance of the context for how the case is initially construed
- with little if any attention to the development of the doctor as a person and a professional.

The deep learning that can come from regular rigorous reflection has not yet been realised by the majority of doctors. They learn little more from 'reflecting on a practice' than is available to them in text books and through discussion in the clinical setting between supervisee and supervisor. Further, since these meet rarely, such learning is highly haphazard!

Transformative Reflection for doctors is not 'a theory' or a protocol to be applied to practice. It is a set of guidelines and prompts to help the learners themselves (whoever they are in the medical hierarchy) to explore and to challenge and critique *their role* and their clinical thinking in a patient case. This is by contrast to how most reflection works in that it uncovers the doctor's contribution to the case, rather than merely reporting the patient's 'pathway' through the case! For the best learning, it does require a wise colleague (for seniors) or a wise supervisor (for doctors in training), to act as further challenger, appreciator or educator, and it does offer broader ways of thinking about each component of clinical practice by indicating wider perspectives on each aspect of the case.

The entire details of TRP have been developed through much direct observation *in situ* of doctors and surgeons at work in practice – sometimes with doctors in training at their side – which has been followed up immediately through deep discussion about the invisible components of that practice, from the doctor's point of view as they engaged with a particular patient case. The understandings derived from this were brought up both to a range of wider educational thinking about the finer details of professional practice, and offered to a wide range of further medical and also senior healthcare professionals. That is: TRP has been theorised from the specifics of a wide range of individual medical practice. (See Fish, 2008.)

The Principles and Components of TRP

For these reasons, we believe that we can claim that the components and processes of medical practice embedded in TRP represent some important elements of what doctors need to be helped to articulate more clearly for the purposes indicated above. We have certainly found that they resonate with over 99% of the practitioners we have offered them to.

The following Table 1.4.1, offers a list of the principles that guide TRP for doctors and the relevant components of medical practice that we derived from our investigations.

Table 1.4.1 The principles and components of TRP

Principles underpinning TRP **The ones in blue are consonant with all reflection**	Components of TRP
Like all practices, TRP must acknowledge the tradition out of which it has been developed	It is a version of Reflective Practice (RP) as offered in Part One of this book and as such it is shaped by all the general principles of RP
It must relate to a theoretical basis	In this case it is related both to the theoretical basis of RP and has arisen through researching and theorising the breadth and depth of the work of doctors and surgeons (see Fish, 2009)
It must be about one's own practice	
It should engage in open-minded enquiry into, and examination of, one's practice	

continued

The anonymity of colleagues, patients and institutions must be preserved

It is, at heart, for professionals, an educational process to which scheduled and recognised time must be given

It must focus on examples of one's own personal practice, carefully selected for their educational potential to illuminate and develop the heart of practice, and not just to explore something that has gone wrong

It should be guided by key prompts about the important components of one's practice, that enable that practice to be unpacked

It should explore various conceptions of professionalism and consider one's own conduct in the light of them

It should utilise all four modes of language (reading, writing, speaking and listening), to support the exploration involved

Detailed writing is itself a means of learning, when it is exploratory. Presentational writing is used in the summary of what has been learnt at the end

Some, but not all writing should be selected to put on record. It should aid the development of a personal vision of professionalism and practice

Everyone needs a 'wise other' to get the best out of the process

For doctors in training it needs to be part of the regularly negotiated Learning Agreement for a clinical attachment

The Essential Resources

1. The starting point of TRP is to make a list of **the bullet points *about the patient's pathway* through the case** (details as at a hand-over)

2. **'The Invisibles'** are the main resource (see de Cossart and Fish, 2005 and Fish and de Cossart, 2007). Each invisible comprises a heuristic and a set of prompts/ questions. The prompts raise questions to consider about each aspect of practice. Each Invisible has its own colour which is used to write about it. These are divided into two groups

The Narrative Invisibles: the context of this case; the person brought to this case; the professional brought to this case; the knowledge brought to this case; the wider view of this case; the therapeutic relationship made with the patient in this case. These enrich the basic clinical story

The interrogative Invisibles: the professional judgements and the clinical decision making made in this case. These aid the unpacking of the underlying nuances of the story

3. **Rainbow Writing**, which is the means of demonstrating the variety of exploration of the piece of practice. Advice is offered in Part Three about a dialogic approach to teaching this

4. **The Final Summary Statement:** derived from the narrative and its interrogation

Chapter Four

Transformative Reflection: how the components interrelate

We offer in Figure 1.4.1 a diagram which interrelates all the elements of the overall process of Transformative Reflection for Doctors.

The line drawing at the centre of the figure puts the vulnerable patient, their loved ones and those who care for them at the heart of this reflection. This central picture is deliberately overlaid by two circles and an oval which overlap each other.

The purple circle represents:

> what we see as the heart of wise practice: the capacity of the doctor to make wise professional judgements underpinned by sound clinical decision making.

The two turquoise circles (of equal size), represent:

1. *The Narrative* of the patient case and what the doctor brought of themselves to the case.
2. *The Exploration of that Narrative* and its interrogation to assess the quality of the doctor's clinical thinking in this case.

The Dark Turquoise Ellipse which overlaps all the others, represents:

> the new understandings and insights that will emerge through what we have now called The Transformative Reflective Process which we describe in more detail below.

Figure 1.4.1 Transformative Reflection for Doctors: How the components interrelate

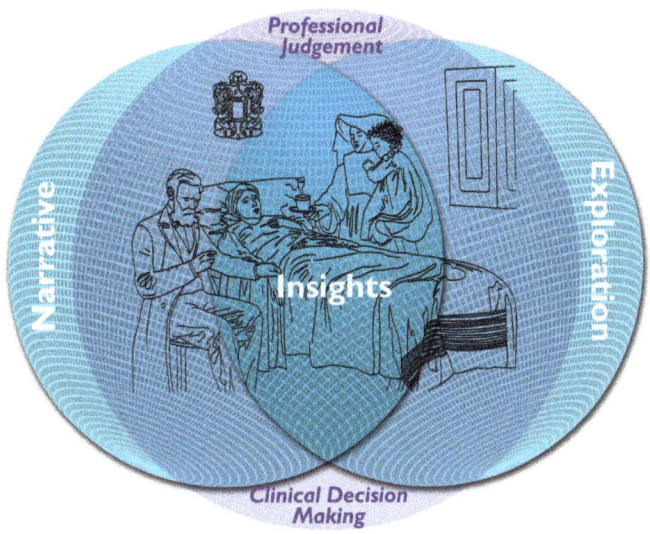

The Transformative Reflective Process in action is shown in Figure 1.4.2 and provided in detail in Part Two.

Figure 1.4.2 Transformative Reflection: The Process

Step One Chapter Five
Selecting the case, developing the bullet points
Outline of a recent case to stimulate thinking and writing
An essential starting point
Moving the focus from the patient to the doctor

Step Two Chapter Six
Creating the narrative
Using the bullet points to create the Doctor-centred narrative
Using *The Invisibles* as prompts and Rainbow Writing
Noting surprising things

Step Three Chapter Seven
Interrogating the case
Exploring and assessing the quality of your Professional Judgements and Clinical Thinking
Noting surprising things

Step Four Chapter Eight
Summarising the results of your efforts
Summarising your new learning
Recording your new understandings and evidence of your development

---

Our educational thinking now underpinning Transformative Reflection

The following provides our refined thinking and understanding of a process that we first began to develop in 2003. It has been informed by our learning as we have taught hundreds of senior doctors and other healthcare professionals over the last sixteen years. As a result of this we have refined and slightly reorganised the processes, components and resources about which we have previously written and placed the emphasis on the transformation of the doctor as learner and the articulation of the qualities of doctors' professionalism, wisdom and moral agency, which need to be shared with the wider world, as argued for in Chapter One.

The construction of and enquiry into the case: a re-vision of the whole enterprise

Our new thinking about reflection for doctors is as follows.

i. Start with the patient and provide and record a skeleton of the patient pathway (which we continue to call the bullet points of the case as before).
ii. Enrich that skeleton with the details of the doctor's perspective (this now involves six narrative Invisibles from the eight we originally invented).
iii. Interrogate the enriched case now containing the patient and the doctor's perspectives (this involves the other two Invisibles we originally invented).
iv. Summarise your learning as the doctor as a result of this process and expect to comment on your professionalism, wisdom and moral agency.

At the end of this process you should think about who you should share this with and to what end.

By seeing this process as a whole in the light of today's needs for the better development of doctors and the better enlightenment of patients, managers and the public, we have turned reflection for doctors into an educational research process, as recommended by Stenhouse (1975).

The following outlines the new process, our reordering of the Invisibles and a reminder of Rainbow Writing which is the best means we have found for capturing and sharing the detail of the complexity of a patient case.

1. The bullet points of the patient case (see Chapter Five)

The starting point for the whole reflective process remains the same as before and requires a carefully chosen case and the chronological ordering of a set of bullet points that chart the key clinical elements of that case. This draws on routine processes very familiar to all doctors for a variety of purposes, where the patient's clinical case is summarised. The bullet points (focused on the patient) offer a scaffold on which to build a much richer narrative which focuses on what the doctor brings to a patient case or event. This stage is represented by the purple circle in Figure 1.4.1.

2. Using what we now call 'The Narrative Invisibles' to enrich the case (See Chapter Six)

The focus of each of the Narrative Invisibles, which should be used in turn, and in the order below, is

- **the context of the chosen case, because this is always unique to a case**
- **the knowledge used by the doctor in the chosen case**
- **the kind of person the doctor brought to the chosen case**
- **the kind of professional the doctor aspires to be in the chosen case**
- **the therapeutic relationship the doctor creates with the patient in the chosen case**
- **the wider perspectives the doctor took into account in that case.**

Different colours are used (as described in Rainbow Writing below) for each invisible which enables the places in which each is found in the narrative, to be identified and considered. This stage is represented by the left hand turquoise circle in Figure 1.4.1 (see p.53).

It omits two key Invisibles from our original list, which now appear below.

3. Using the Exploratory Invisibles (see Chapter Seven)

The enriched narrative then becomes the focus for interrogation of what we see as the heart of wise practice, that is, the professional judgements made throughout the case and the process of decision making that led to them.

These Invisibles explore the quality of clinical thinking and have been created from our Clinical Thinking Pathway. We have called them:

- **Invisible Seven: Professional Judgement** which explores the quality of professional judgements leading to the key actions;
- **Invisible Eight: Clinical decision making** which unpicks the type of clinical decision making (clinical reasoning or deliberation) which informed those professional judgements.

4. Creating a summary that distills your new learning (see Chapter Eight)

The thoughtful and in-depth exploration of the qualities and capacities that the doctor brings to a patient case, unpacked at step two and three of The Transformative Reflective

Process, will produce the evidence of new insights that underpin the new learning and deeper thinking revealed. The summary will only be the headlines of the insights arising from this deeper learning and will be a pointer to the need for further professional development and changes in practice. This stage is represented by the dark turquoise ellipse in Figure 1.4.1.

The Summary cannot be created until the end of the process. It is the public surface/product of a great depth of learning as revealed when working through the whole of the TRP. It is often the only thing required in official documents, missing the point that both product and process are extremely valuable.

Over the years of teaching reflective writing in seminars, we have been robustly challenged about the writing that you are learning to do here. Typical comments we have received include: *I cannot write so it will be very difficult for me! Why is it necessary to write so much? I don't think I will have enough to say.* No one who we personally have taught in a seminar has been unable to write and all have realised great insights as they have worked through the process for themselves. The learning is in the writing (Fish and Coles, 1998).

Postscript to this section

Sometimes the narrative itself should be shared. This is particularly the case in teaching supervisees. It may even be something that occasionally (and for the right reasons), is shared with patients, managers and others. Whatever stage of expertise the doctor is at, the powerful impact of a series of cases treated in this way will build a picture of the development and quality of the practice of that doctor.

The Narrative and Exploratory Invisibles

The Invisibles were conceived by the authors in 2003, following a time of researching and unpacking what a doctor (in this case a surgeon) calls upon in their everyday clinical practice as they make professional judgements. The quality of those judgements are what define the quality and wisdom of the doctor (de Cossart and Fish, 2005; Fish and de Cossart, 2007; Fish and de Cossart, 2013).

Figure 1.4.3 shows each of our eight Invisibles, their memorable Heuristic and their Reflective Focus. It is followed by a short comment about each.

Figure 1.4.3 The Invisibles, their Heuristic and their Reflective Focus

The Narrative Invisibles

The Invisible	Heuristic	Reflective Focus
Context	Woman under Willows	The importance of the context of the case or event and the **interpretations made about it** cannot be overstated.
Kind of person you are	Iceberg	This is about one's **personal values / assumptions / beliefs** as related to the case or event.
Kind of professional you are	Continuum — Extended / Restricted	This is about exploring **one's professionalism** in relation to the case or event.

Chapter Four

The Invisible	Heuristic	Reflective Focus
14 Forms of Knowledge	**Knowledge Cards**	This is the **range** and **kinds of knowledge** one brings to the case.
The Therapeutic Relationship	**Doctor with Patient**	This shows the **quality of the relationship created between doctor and the patient.**
Contextual awareness	**Faded out background**	This involves **seeing beyond the case** and all that is going on in its background and the wider global context of practice.

The Exploratory Invisibles

The Invisible	Heuristic	Reflective Focus
Professional Judgement	CTP 1 Decisions to Act	This is the **quality of professional judgement** both *personal* and *product* one brings to a case.
Clinical Decision-making	CTP 2 Thinking processes underlying the decision to act	This is the complex pathway of **one's clinical reasoning and deliberation**.

Please note the colours in column three mirror the rainbow writing colours as set out on pages 53 & 64.

A short comment about each of our eight Invisibles

Each of *The Invisibles* also has an heuristic (a memorable picture) and a reflective focus which is what is being explored in talking or writing reflectively when prompted by ideas related to that particular Invisible. You will see for yourself how this works in Chapters Six and Seven. Here we offer a brief summary.

The Narrative Invisibles

Context

The Heuristic for *Context* is a picture developed from Monet's 'Woman under Willows'. A print of the original work, (Monet, 1880), was hanging on the wall of a room in which we were first writing about this topic. An embellished sketch became our heuristic to remind us that everything is affected by how we 'read' the context in which an event occurs, and that how we understand that context will seriously colour our interpretation of that event and our response to it.

The Reflective Focus here is the interpretation about the patient case that is always made by the doctor and which is very likely to affect both their judgements and their underpinning thinking for both diagnosis and treatment.

The Iceberg of Practice

The Heuristic, *The Iceberg of Practice* (Fish and Coles, 1998) was adapted to remind us that what is observed of the actions of a doctor is only a very small part of what is going on in the mind of the doctor. The Reflective Focus here is to explore in a given case how the tacit elements influence the doctor's actions particularly their personal values, assumptions and beliefs. These colour the kind of person we are as a doctor and what we bring (to some extent variably) to meeting and caring for each specific patient. It is also salutary to remember that patients are often very sharp at reading the tacit beneath our surface!

Professionalism

The Heuristic here is the Extended and Restricted Professional (E/R) table. It builds on the work of Hoyle (Hoyle, 1974). The paired statements in each row represent the beginning and end of a continuum related to an aspect of our professionalism, and are not intended to be an 'either/or' descriptor, but to provoke thought about how one conducted oneself as a medical professional, in a particular case. You will meet this in detail in Chapter Six. The Reflective focus here is the exploration of the kind of professional that you brought (or didn't bring) to the specific case being reflected on.

The Forms of Knowledge

The Heuristic here is fourteen 'playing cards' arranged in a Y shape, which were created to show our fourteen forms of the kinds of knowledge a doctor may draw upon during a particular case. The Reflective Focus here is to explore the range and kind of knowledge that doctors bring to the case which usually goes well beyond the textbook knowledge and visible skills. Most clinical case discussions, never explore these and so many learning opportunities are therefore lost.

The Therapeutic Relationship

A print entitled 'Science and Charity' (Picasso, 1897) hangs on Linda's office wall, and was chosen as the Heuristic for considering the therapeutic relationship the doctor makes with a patient. It artistically and compassionately encapsulates the vulnerability of the patient, and those around her. It emphasises the unique (and expert) position of the doctor in this relationship.

The reflective focus here is on the quality of the relationship created between the doctor and the patient. We reserve the term 'therapeutic' for the very special relationship that indicates the mutual *working together* of a wise doctor who brings a range of qualities and a patient who is willing not merely to meet the doctor, but where appropriate to reveal to the doctor 'the particularity of their case and the individuality of their being'. Such a 'willingness', depends more on how the doctor meets the patient, than on the character of the patient, (Campbell, 1984).

Contextual Awareness

The Heuristic here shows two similar photographs of an operating scene, one of which has been adjusted to put the background in outline only, the other has the background in colour and focus.

The reflective focus here is to explore what doctors see and is aware of beyond the immediacy of the case in front of them. Doctors who are relatively new to medical practice focus almost exclusively on the immediate circle of their own activities (and those of their clinical supervisor). They are not even aware of what occurs at the periphery of their vision. Thus learning to practise with greater maturity is about becoming aware of the wider view and drawing it more into focus. In order to 'see' as their expert senior colleagues see, doctors must learn the habit of looking with 'a discerning eye' (Fish, 1998). It has been compared with, and has some resonance with, what others have called situational awareness (Yule et al., 2006).

The Exploratory Invisibles

Professional Judgement

Clinical Thinking Pathway 1 (CTP1) is the Heuristic for the professional judgements that a doctor makes throughout the process of caring for a patient. The purple colours within the heuristic indicate a) the personal professional judgements (made at various stages *on the way to* the main decision about the treatment of the patient), these are often binary and routine; and b) the final product professional judgement, the 'final' decision that prefigures the major action (the ultimate treatment of the patient, or at least the climax of a major stage of the patient's treatment). The reflective focus of this is to sharpen the doctor's awareness of the many decisions they make during a case and to scrutinise them for their quality. This Invisible is the first of the exploratory Invisibles (See more in Chapter Seven.)

Clinical Decision Making

Clinical Thinking Pathway 2 (CTP2) is the Heuristic for the clinical decision making (the various shades of turquoise-green in the model) that underpins the professional judgements made in a case by the doctor. They may be compared to the often invisible 'workings out' of a complex mathematical calculation which should explains how the answer was reached.

The turquoise-green colours represent at the top end of the clinical thinking pathway the more scientific/formulaic decisions which we refer to as clinical reasoning, where the doctor collects evidence about 'the patient's case' and reasons about it scientifically, leading to a focused clinical diagnosis and a solution that is the *right* one generally for such a case. In contrast, we see the more humanistic bottom end of the pathway, represented by the darker green colour, which we characterise as deliberation, where all the doctor's thinking is driven, not by what is right for such a case generally (wherever it is found), but by a concern for what is *best* for this particular patient who has individual needs.

The reflective focus here is to make this thinking, which is usually tacit and unexplored, explicit and therefore able to be interrogated for its quality and appropriateness. It is quite impossible to make a self-assessment of one's own practice without doing this. *Without sharing such thinking, with young learners, the nuances and complexities of practice will take longer to be learned and embedded in practice.*

Rainbow Writing

This development of a way of teaching medical reflective writing was created by Della. Each of the eight elements shown in Figure 1.4.3 have a colour associated with them. The particular colours for each of the elements were arbitrary but now have become set for this particular process of learning the technique.

An early cohort of Masters students christened it as *Rainbow Writing*. They offered very helpful critique of the process and used this with their trainees in parallel with their own learning of it. None were more surprised than each of them how enthusiastic the trainees they engage with were about doing it. They learned too that when starting to use the process it is better to explore only two Invisibles at a time. This makes the process more manageable, in terms of time and preparation. Learning any new process always takes longer than those experienced in it ultimately need.

This technique of *Rainbow Writing* we will encourage you to use later on in the book. The colours work both to remind you of what element you are writing about and when the writing is complete as a diagnostic visual aid of what elements were most involved in the thinking in the case. In classroom seminar teaching we use pens, pencils and paper but for personal use the computer and word processing works well too. Our publication *Reflection for Medical Appraisal (2013)*, is to date the most detailed description of how to create a piece of *Rainbow Writing* and then to interrogate it to explore the quality of clinical thinking in a particular patient case or event. It expands on the way to use *The Invisibles* and *Rainbow Writing* for the specific purposes of appraisal and how they help a clinician to link their exploration to the requirements of the GMC. We have used this book as a guide for over thirty, one-day workshops, on *Reflection for Medical Appraisal* sharing it with nearly five hundred senior doctors across the specialities of medicine. It has been well received. The following figure 1.4.4 offers a reminder of the colours now traditionally used for Rainbow Writing.

Figure 1.4.4   Rainbow Writing Colours

The colours now used in this process are:

BLACK   the bullet points outlining your case

The Narrative Colours
Blue 1   the **CONTEXT** of this particular case
Blue 2   the **KIND OF PERSON** you brought to the case
Green   the **PROFESSIONALISM** you brought to the case
Red   the **FORMS OF KNOWLEDGE** you brought to the case
Pink   the **THERAPEUTIC RELATIONSHIP** with the patient
Turquoise   **WIDER CONTEXTUAL AWARENESS** in the case

The Exploratory Colours
Brown   Professional Judgement
Purple   Clinical Reasoning and Deliberation

Endnote

The next four chapters will guide you carefully through the Transformative Reflective Process. You will need to have chosen a suitable patient case.

Part Two

Transformative Reflection: The process and methodology

Introduction to Part Two

Transformative Reflective Writing is both patient centred and doctor centred. It offers a sound educationally focused reflective process specifically designed to help all doctors develop themselves as people and practitioners. Its intentions are to nurture the doctor in becoming a better doctor preparing them to be able to offer better patient care.

Part Two offers our refined process of Reflective Writing for doctors as set out in The Transformative Reflective Pathway. (See Figure 1.4.2), using Rainbow Writing. Each step is described in detail in the chapters that follow. As you become familiar with the process, these steps will become second nature. The process described in this part is focused on senior doctors because it is important that those who will both model its use and teach it, are proficient and confident with doing so. Part Three will concentrate on teaching this to others.

Chapter Five will take you through Step One of the Transformative Reflective Process and guide you through selecting your case and developing the bullet points. We strongly recommend that you use a case of your own and work through the exercise for yourself. This will give you the most authentic feel for what is happening during the activity.

Chapter Six offers the steps for creating a reflective narrative of your patient case or event.

Chapter Seven describes the process of interrogating the narrative to explore the qualities of clinical thinking you used in this case.

Chapter Eight will guide the summarising of your new understandings, accrued through the process, and pinpoint the evidence that has led to this.

By the end of Part Two you will have your first draft of your written reflective account of what you consciously or subconsciously, brought to bear on your clinical thinking in your chosen case. The process of creating this rich narrative may prompt surprises or new insights. You are encouraged to make a note of these as you go, they will be part of your new understanding that will emerge through this activity. The completed and refined narrative is the focus for you to explore and examine your professional judgements, their underlying clinical reasoning.

A series of cases and/or events written in this way will build a rich picture of your growing professional identity and expertise as a physician or surgeon.

Chapter Five

Prioritising time, selecting the case and developing the bullet points

> Introduction
> Prioritising time for learning this new activity
> Wise case selection: being alert to the educational opportunities
> The implications of writing digitally or by hand
> Creating the Bullet Points
> An example of a set of bullets
> Endnote

Introduction

Take this chapter seriously because failure to start in the right place will hinder your progress. It emphasises the importance of prioritising time for learning this new activity because being a Reflective Practitioner is a key marker of being a good professional. This chapter highlights the importance of wise case selection that is appropriate to the context of your experience, and describes creating the bullet points to facilitate the reflective process. It emphasises the need for accuracy and thoroughness of the bullet points with respect to the clinical details of the patient's case. It will prepare you to go on to stage two where you use the six Narrative Invisibles to prompt the development of your account to focus on what you brought to the case, and stage three where you interrogate the full case to reveal your professional judgements and clinical thinking.

The bulleted outline is the usual way of charting the patient case for practical purposes in everyday medical practice. When you have finally completed the whole narrative process at the end of stage three, you will be surprised how minimalistic the original bullet point outline was in representing the complexity of your own thinking and actions within this case.

Prioritising time for learning this new activity

To practice as a doctor cannot be learned from a text book. The huge depth of thinking that underlies your practical clinical experience will only transform into a deep understanding of it and of yourself as a practitioner, through rigorous reflection on that experience. We believe that quiet space and time spent thoughtfully in well-focused reflection will both sharpen your thinking and the quality of your practice and, perhaps more valuably, invigorate you as a practitioner.

We encourage you, when you begin this whole process, to schedule time and space in your diary for learning this method. It may seem slow to start with but as you become familiar with the process it will become second nature. Doing this is a very appropriate use of *Supporting Professional Activities* (SPA) time, or of personal study leave. Research has shown this learning experience to be educationally worthwhile Thomé, (2012; 2013); Bullock et al, (2012); and Fish, (2012). It should be fun too, and the things you learn about yourself and your practice should be emancipatory and transformative, leading to new thinking and new ideas for your professional life.

Wise case selection: being alert to the educational opportunities

The wise choice of a case for reflection is essential. It will depend on your seniority and your experience and expertise as a physician or surgeon. We advise, whilst you are learning this process, that you explore cases that are not involved in controversy. Such cases introduce an added emotional burden to learning a new method which will become a hindrance. Choose a case that is relatively straightforward. Ordinary everyday cases will offer you much more than at first you might think! As you become more confident with the method, then you can increase the complexity of the case chosen.

The chosen case for this exercise should then, in principle be:

- one where you, the doctor, has had significant responsibility in caring for the patient
- one where you yourself have made a range of key decisions about the patient's treatment
- current and interesting for you
- relevant to your capacity and expertise as a physician or surgeon
- likely to contain learning opportunities for your development as a clinician or a teacher.

The choice of case as a consultant and senior doctor

Consultants and senior doctors may engage in the discipline of reflective practice for some of the following reasons:

- for their own interest in clarifying thinking and exploring in depth a particular case from their practice
- as a means of unearthing their own clinical thinking in preparation for case discussion at grand rounds, talking to patients and their relatives, talking to their clinical team about specific cases and events, and for presenting lines of argument for actions taken, to peers, experts and the public at large
- for considering how your own practice offers learning opportunities to respond to the GMC's requirement to teach *Generic Professional Capabilities*, because TRP offers you a way of exploring for yourself, your professional values and behaviours, your professional skills and your professional knowledge, through specific case study

- in order to give you the experience to teach this process to supervisees.

We stress that the activity is not aimed at finding out just what went well or what went badly in the case. The main transforming effect of reflective practice will be:

- a deepening understanding about the complexities of your thought and actions in your practice
- an appreciation of your current level of expertise
- a realisation of how you may work to develop and strengthen yourself in being a doctor
- a vocabulary and logic to explain better what you did and why, to any who may need to know.

Cases explored on paper through TRP, when carefully filed and stored, will over time be a rich source of evidence to demonstrate your development and growth as a medical practitioner. This will also be a rich resource for teaching opportunities. Your professional discipline in creating and keeping these records will model good professional practice to young doctors. It will be a resource that may be shared with patients and others to demonstrate your commitment to professionalism, wisdom and moral agency.

As your confidence and experience develops with this process, you may choose to use it to respond to situations of dispute and complaint. It is very useful for this. It will be important however, not to use the process to 'show off'.

The implications of writing digitally or by hand

Although there is no absolute right or wrong, there are some important points to consider in choosing which method you use to write. Some of the most important guiding principles are as follows.

- Writing slows down the mind and gives more time to think as you write. It is often this process that sparks new insights which are the beginning of transformations of thinking.
- Using paper and pencil allows creative linking of ideas and concepts which may be refined later on a digital medium, but are often rather more technically difficult to capture straight onto a computer.
- Availability of and ability to use the digital equipment must not interfere with either the educational intention of the activity or the fluidity of the process.
- Digital writing may be more appropriate to parts of the process than others. For example a pen and paper is often more useful in starting and brainstorming ideas which may then be digitally refined later.

Creating the Bullet Points

The creation of a clinically accurate set of bullet points about the patient case is essential if your reflection is to begin well. It can become a useful starting point for reflecting on the case by taking each bullet point in turn, because it takes away the heart-sink feeling of facing a blank piece of paper and also it is the scaffold on which the rest of the process builds.

Writing the bullet points should take the format of what you might create as a timeline of what happened to the patient during a particular illness, for the purposes of a clinical presentation at a multidisciplinary meeting (MDT) or a Grand Round. It will contain the order of events, the facts and results of tests that the patient underwent. It is patient focused and rarely contains elaborate detail of what the doctor brought of themselves and their expertise to the clinical case. In usual clinical conversations in practice the thinking behind the facts is rarely made explicit and explored and is not captured for detailed re-consideration.

As in any written account of a patient's case, anonymity must be attended to. Names of patients and doctors must not appear. This must be double checked if the reflection is to be uploaded as part of an educational or an appraisal portfolio.

An example of a set of bullets

Figure 2.5.1 shows a typical example of a series of bullet points captured in preparation for beginning TRP. It is particularly useful to note that the patient's care is (appropriately) the focus of this and the patient is properly anonymised. You will see by the end of the next chapter how little evidence there is of what the doctor brought to the case.

Figure 2.5.1 Bullet points of a consultant case.

- A 49-year-old female librarian was referred to me because of a persistent discharge from her left ear.

- Clinical examination revealed granulomatous disease in a tympanic membrane retraction pocket.

- The patient was referred for a CT scan, which confirmed the presence of cholesteatoma.

- At the clinic following the scan, I explained the findings of the scan; namely disease in the left ear (which had poor levels of hearing), but was the patient's only hearing ear.

- I discussed with one of my colleagues about proceeding with surgery on the left ear, and with another colleague about what options were available for the patient if she did go deaf in the left ear after surgery.

- I then met the patient again in the outpatient department. She was extremely anxious to go ahead with surgery as she had already spent a lot of time off work because of the condition. I agreed and the decision was made to proceed with the operation.

- During the operation on the left ear I removed the disease from the attic region of the ear but was left with the dilemma about removing the pocket over the stapes (the third hearing bone). I left the pocket undisturbed.

- At one-month post-operation the patient was recovering well from her surgery.

Endnote

Now you need to select your case and prepare your bullet points. Having done this, you are ready to continue on to the next chapter.

Chapter Six

Transformative Reflective Writing: Creating the doctor-centred narrative

Introduction
Creating your narrative using The Narrative Invisibles and their Prompts
Refining Your First Draft
An example of Rainbow Writing by a consultant surgeon
Endnote

Introduction

This chapter falls into three main sections. It first guides you through the process of using the Narrative Invisibles with the bullets of the patient case to build a narrative about **what you the doctor** brought to the case. This exploration and development is at the heart of what the General Medical Council is trying to develop in their *Generic Professional Capabilities Framework* (2019). The second section offers ways of refining your writing to sharpen the focus of the account. The chapter ends with an opportunity to see an example of rainbow writing from a consultant surgeon who was once one of our Masters students.

Doctors write prolifically as part of their professional life. Do not be doubtful about your abilities in this activity. Where the writing you usually do is about 'someone else' and at 'arms-length', here you will be writing about yourself, which at first may seem a little uncomfortable but you might find that actually this is easier. Remember that reflection is about understanding yourself better, to be able to develop and grow as a person and a doctor. We have yet to meet a doctor who cannot engage with this. If you are careful to follow in order what is offered in this chapter you will find that your narrative will emerge.

General Points

Your starting point is to take the list of your bullet points outlining your patient case which you created in response to Chapter Five. Use more bullet points to respond to the prompts in each of the narrative Invisibles as you build the content of your narrative. You will be encouraged to create flowing prose (proper sentences and paragraphs in a logical order). Later, when you redraft the piece you will of course very quickly find your own voice once you have begun.

We stress here at the beginning, that the prompts accompanying *The Invisibles* are not a protocol list to be followed slavishly but are there to help to stimulate your thinking about your part in the case. There may be some prompts that are simply not relevant for your particular case. Please remember to anonymise any names of the patient and any staff who were part of the case.

We teach you to use the Rainbow Writing Colours for expanding your narrative and Figure 2.6.1 below reminds you of the font colours for each of the Narrative Invisibles. The colours were chosen arbitrarily but are now fixed by traditional use.

Figure 2.6.1   *Rainbow Writing Colours for building the narrative*

The colours to be used in this process are:

Black	**the bullet points outlining your case**
Blue 1	the **CONTEXT** of this particular case
Blue 2	the **KIND OF PERSON** you brought to the case
Green	the **PROFESSIONALISM** you brought to the case
Red	the **FORMS OF KNOWLEDGE** you brought to the case
Pink	the **THERAPEUTIC RELATIONSHIP** with the patient
Turquoise	your **WIDER CONTEXTUAL AWARENESS** in the case

See page 64

Chapter Six

Creating your narrative using The Narrative Invisibles and their Prompts

Preparing the Bullet points to start writing

- Writing on computer or on paper, put the date and Draft One at the top of your first page, insert page numbers.
- List your bullet points created in Chapter Five, below this heading. Leave space at the top for the title of your completed writing which will emerge as your writing progresses.
- Next take a copy of each of your bullet points and put one bullet point at the top of each of a new page keeping the chronological order you first created. Use as many pages as you have bullet points.
- Then, as you continue through the chapter, for each bullet point work through the prompts for each of the six Narrative Invisible that follow and, use the appropriate font colour for each Invisibles to record your list of relevant responses to the prompts. By this method you will begin to make explicit those responses and what lay behind them in this patient case.

Now you will start to enrich your bullet points using the Narrative Invisibles.

You might find tackling no more than two Invisibles at a time, the most manageable.

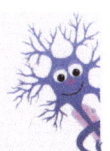

Transformative Reflection for Practicing Physicians and Surgeons

Invisible 1: Context BLUE

Figure 2.6.2 The Context Heuristic

Our version of a Monet painting to prompt a recognition of the **Interpretations** registered early in the case

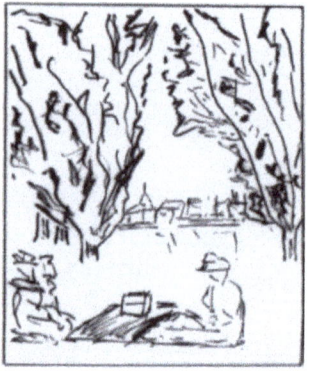

Every patient case is unique. The importance of context of a case and how this shapes the unquestioned interpretations made about the whole case by the doctor, cannot be overstated. The contextual elements you see and hear whenever you meet a patient are liable to affect both your judgement and the underpinning thinking that will go into both the diagnosis and the quality of the treatment offered.

Use the prompts below to expand your writing. Add your own questions if you feel there is something missing. Consider the prompts in relation to each of your bullet points. Not all will need further expansion. Remember to write in Blue.

The Prompts

Ask as many of the following questions as are appropriate for your case.

- How did you get to know about the case (who told you and how did they tell you)?
- What were the significant factors related to the time and circumstances of your first (and any later) meeting(s) with this patient?
- What did you particularly notice about the physical environment at the time?
- What other contextual matters were significant to you?
- Say something about the individual patient:
  - how they presented at your first meeting
  - what their body language told you
  - what you sensed about how the patient saw themselves in relation to their medical problem
  - how the environment influenced your inter-relations and your thinking (was the meeting in the patient's own environment or yours?)
  - was there anything significant about the order in which the patient presented information?
  - was there anything significant in what was not said?
- were there any cultural, social, or community issues that were tacit beneath the surface?
- who else was there, what difference did this make (what did they introduce

into the scene, and why, or what was that a result of)?
- how did all this affect your understanding / interpretation of the case?

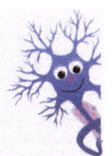

*Did anything surprise you about what you have added into the case narrative?
If so, make a note ready for use in Chapter Eight.*

Transformative Reflection for Practicing Physicians and Surgeons

Invisible 2: The kind of person you brought to the case BLUE

Figure 2.6.3 The Iceberg Heuristic

(modified from Fish and Coles, 1998, see also Fish, 2015)

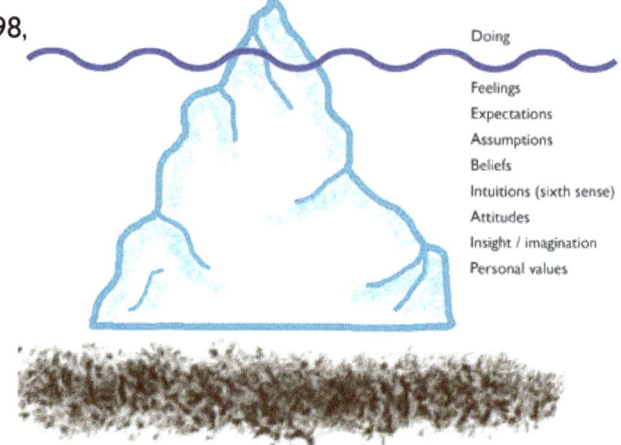

As you come to meet a patient, person to person, your invisible personal virtues, values, assumptions and beliefs will shape that meeting and your explicit conduct will reveal in your actions and body language how you relate to the patient and their case. This is often what a patient will remember about you. No inauthentic behaviour adopted for the moment will dupe a discerning patient or for that matter other colleagues, about who you are as a medical professional. Knowing yourself is a very important strength.

The Iceberg Heuristic (Figure 2.6.3) reminds us that what is visible in practice (above the water) is only a very small part of the whole person the doctor is. In your case, your personal values, assumptions, beliefs, expectations, attitudes, intuitions and feelings will have influenced your decision making. It is not by chance that your personal values are at the broad foundation of the iceberg. Your personal values are a strong influence on how you see the world.

Consider the following about yourself in this case. Each point needs to be attended to.

Your Feelings
Don't ignore any relevant emotions that you may have felt about the case and its context, they were part of the scene however well you disguised them (for example: irritation at something; pleasure in meeting this patient).

Your Expectations
What were you expecting the patient to be like / to need / to be suffering from and did you have to adjust these expectations in the light of reality?

Your Assumptions
What did you assume about the patient or the case at first meeting? Were you right? What had fuelled your assumptions?

Your Beliefs
What beliefs of yours about the patient, the case, the disease and how you see the world, were challenged or were reinforced by this case?

Your Intuitions
What role (if any) did your intuition play in this case? How did such intuition arise? Was it correct?

Your Attitudes
What was your attitude to the patient? Did something get between you and seeing them fully? Or did your attitude to them obscure your view of something?

Your Insight / imagination
How did you understand how the patient saw themselves and their problems and / or the possible solutions? Did you even consider this?

Your Personal values
What personal priorities shaped how you conducted yourself in the case? What personal priorities did you suppress in this case and why?

*Again make a note of anything that surprised you in doing this writing.
If so make a note ready for use in Chapter Eight.*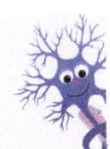

Transformative Reflection for Practicing Physicians and Surgeons

Invisible 3: The kind of Professional you brought to the case   GREEN

Figure 2.6.4 The Extended/Restricted Professional Continuum Heuristic

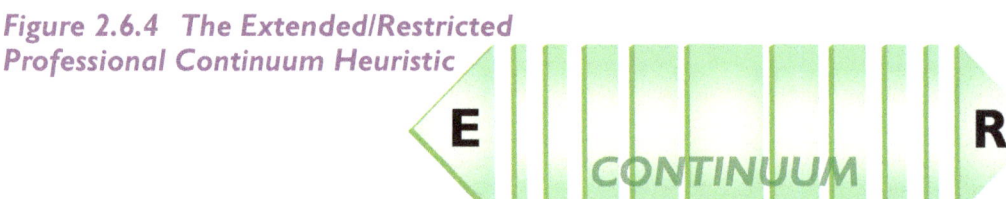

Patients, as well as doctors themselves, have their own ideas of the kind of professional a doctor should be. Because doctors are human beings, however, what a doctor actually brings to a given case, in terms of their professionalism, though dependable, is variable rather than unchanging, and is affected by a wide range of influencing factors that are specific to the day. Also, the nature of each patient will demand different professional responses. The grid below offers some ideas of how one's professionalism might look. Despite aiming to be the best professional possible we don't often achieve this. Consider your professionalism in relation to this particular case. You might place yourself anywhere along the continuum indicated from extended to restricted professional. Look carefully at the grid and then respond to the prompts below.

Figure 2.6.5 The Extended/Restricted Professional Grid
Significantly adapted from Fish and de Cossart, 2007. p. 86

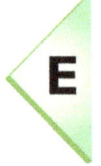 Sees the expertise of a doctor as developed through experience, reading and reflection

Sees the expertise of the doctor as simply defined by the contractual obligations of their employment

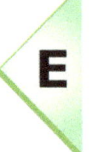 Sees the nature of clinical practice as eternally evolving, which requires a problem-solving approach and educational development especially in respect of professional judgement

Expects the detail and nature of clinical practice to be laid down by outside agencies, which requires the application of protocols through training

Sees the doctor as bringing everything they can offer to the therapeutic and holistic care of the specific patient

Sees the doctor almost exclusively in terms of their technical competence and specialist knowledge in respect of a part of a patient's body

Chapter Six

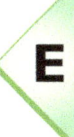 Engages in practical reasoning in which all knowledge, thought processes, actions, and personal attributes are harnessed in the service of the individual patient's case

Engages in technical reasoning and rule following which requires objectivity, and absolves the doctor from engaging in complex thinking and using professional judgement so often R

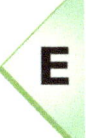 Recognises that practice is interpretive and that a doctor's own values and philosophy will inevitably colour that interpretation

Considers practice to be based on objective knowledge and does not see the significance to practice of own professional values and philosophy R

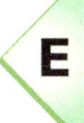 Sees medical practice as a moral enterprise

Does not focus on the moral obligations of clinical practice R

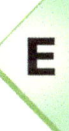 Understands that the wisdom of medical practice is dependent on the quality of the professional judgements made on the spot in relation to the given context

Does not value professional judgement. Values only what can be measured. R

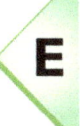 Sees accountability as giving an account of the choices available and made, in a given situation, and the personal philosophy that drove these

Sees accountability as about conformity to the requirements of external authority, which excludes choice, and simply requires rules to be followed. R

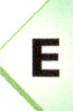 Concerned with long- as well as short-term goals and considers wider social context and later times. Places value on professional collaboration and development at local and national level

Only interested in short term goals — survival and getting on with the job. See clinical events in isolation from each other and ignores the significance of any wider perspectives and professional development R

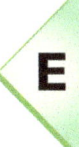 Reads frequently in a wide range of literature relevant to professional practice generally

Derides reading as something active practitioners do not need and do not have time to try to understand R

83

Some questions to consider

- Ask yourself as a professional *in this case*: did I, in general, take:

  an over-broad view of this case
  or a narrow and restricted one
  or was I somewhere near the ideal kind of professional here that the best would aspire to?

- Did I expect this case to be simpler than it was or did I expect it to be more complex than it turned out to be, or did I see the case accurately from the start?

- Did I engage in a problem-solving approach to what the case needed, or did I rely solely on protocols, or did I take a pragmatic approach, using both appropriately?

- Did I consider the whole patient, or merely treat the disease, or consider both appropriately?

- Did I draw only on my technical expertise as a doctor/surgeon (using my skills and technical knowledge alone), or did I go with my heart, humanity and instincts, or did I engage both in the service of the patient?

- Did I engage in technical logic alone, or humane judgement alone or practical reasoning using both?

- Was I over sensitive to the moral and ethical issues here or blind to them, or did I simply seek the best course of action for the patient?

- Was I concerned with only the short-term goals for the patient, or only the long-term goals or both?

- Do I regularly seek further professional development geared to improving my practice or do I see further professional development as a good way of having an easy day? (or both?)

*What other questions and thoughts are springing into your mind as you do this writing?
Make a note ready for use in Chapter Eight.*

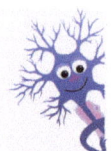

Chapter Six

Transformative Reflection for Practicing Physicians and Surgeons

Invisible 4: The Knowledge cards RED

Figure 2.6.6 The Knowledge Heuristic

Affected and shaped by values, and always context specific to the clinical setting

Procedural Knowledge
Skills, know-how, processes, procedures (related to clinical; managerial; educational; research matters at Trust-level)

Propositional Knowledge
Formal specialist theory, formal generic theory, knowledge of context, of education, of managment, of organization, of profession, of society

Procedural Improvisation Knowledge
How to use and adapt know-how safely to the given context

Evidence Based Knowledge
Knowledge of all appropriate research as relevant

Propositional Adaptation Knowledge
Knowing how to reorganize factual knowledge/skills to respond to the given case

Metacognitive Knowledge
Knowledge of the structure of knowledge and higher order ways of organizing knowing

Professional Knowledge and Conduct
Knowledge of the traditions and parameters of the practice of the profession and its legal framework

Experiential Knowledge
Knowledge gained from undergoing experiences and reflecting on them to make sense of them and learn from them

Practice Generated Knowledge
New knowledge created through undertaking, exploring, and theorizing an aspect of professional practice (can lead to new propositional and procedural knowledge)

Ethical Knowledge
Knowledge of ethical and moral principles that guide all professional practice and that will shape the safe improvisation of procedural knowledge and the re-organization of propositional knowledge

Sensory Knowledge
All that knowledge, both procedural and propositional that comes to the practitioner through their senses

Self Knowledge
Accurate knowledge of own personal characteristics, values and beliefs, plus procedural capabilities and grasp of propositional knowledge

Intuitive Knowledge
Something that we know or are moved to do but cannot (yet) give logical or evidential grounds for

Insight / Imagination
A sudden holistic grasp of an aspect of procedural, propositional or self-knowledge, or knowledge of others

de Cossart and Fish, 2005

Chapter Six

The knowledge a doctor brings to a case includes both propositional knowledge (facts or 'knowing that') and skills (or knowing 'how to'). We do not underestimate the importance of these, which is why they are at the top of our cards, opposite. However, the forms of knowledge you bring to a patient case will be far more than the textbook empirical knowledge and visible skills that you have learned. We have described fourteen forms of knowledge to help a clinical teacher 'diagnose' what 'knowing' they have called upon (or in some cases should have called upon). (See de Cossart and Fish, 2005, Fish and de Cossart, 2007 and 2013.)

So, what do you think of this idea that there is more to knowledge than the textbook and the skills we use? How do you see the knowledge you draw on in a case? In considering this you will not only be exploring your case but also developing your language on how to talk about medical knowledge to patients, colleagues and those you teach. Use the knowledge heuristic on the opposite page to help you identify the knowledge you drew on as the doctor in your case. You may not be adding much more here but highlighting what you have already written and now recatagorising it as a different Invisible, by changing its colour.

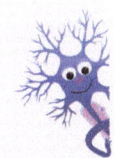

**How many different forms of knowledge did you use in your case?
What surprised you in doing this?
Make a note ready for use in Chapter Eight.**

Invisible 5: The Therapeutic Relationship PINK

Figure 2.6.7 The Therapeutic Relationship Heuristic

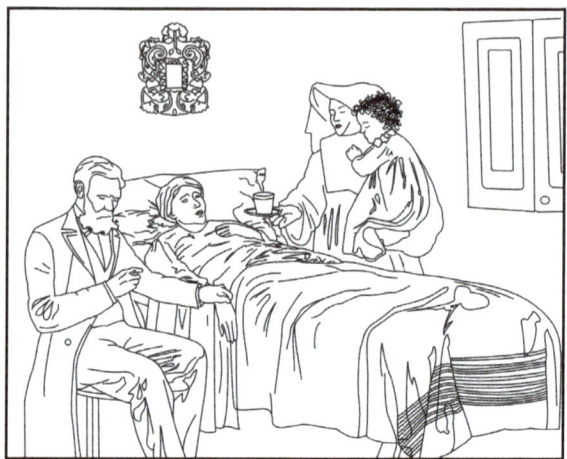

We offer here a line drawing of a Picasso painting (Science and Charity, 1897) of a very sick patient with her doctor, with those who care for her and those who love her and we offer some writing on patients' vulnerabilities. We invite you to attend carefully to the picture and the following words to begin to think more deeply and at the level of principle, about the doctor/patient relationship you sought to achieve in your case.

Our Comments on the Doctor/Patient Relationship

The doctor in the picture is gently considering the context and examining the patient. In the original painting the patient looks very ill. We can only imagine the rest. The inclusion of a child at the bedside of a very sick woman is rather modern by the standards of the day. Perhaps this is Picasso indicating to us the importance of not excluding key members of the family. (Fish and de Cossart, 2007.)

Patients are vulnerable. No matter how much they know about themselves, their symptoms and sometimes their diagnosis, they have to have doctors to confirm their disease, to offer them treatment and to provide 'not simply presence but skill, not just personal concern but highly disciplined services targeted on specific needs' (William F May, quoted in Campbell, 1984: 92).

However strong patients are in their suffering, it usually reduces their stamina and weakens their belief in themselves. By contrast, doctors are powerful as result of their skills and knowledge. They are expected to have physical strength and staying power; and they are highly motivated to cure, improve or, at minimum, palliate, the sick. But their sense that they can almost always improve the lot of the patient, can seduce some doctors into enjoying the exercise of their power. Is there a slight but significant balance to be kept between caring as a selfless service to others (insofar as we humanly can) and caring for the sick as a means of being – or of demonstrating that one is –

virtuous. And is one being 'virtuous' for the sake of the patient or for the privilege and power that virtue brings?

The aspect of medicine that we are encouraging you to explore here is about a less calculating and more humanistic approach to the patient. A doctor's ability to create a nurturing relationship (or not) with their patients will shape the patient's experience and the doctor's whole professional life, making it meaningful or leaving it devoid of something inexpressible yet significant.

By 'the therapeutic relationship' then, we mean something special about the way the doctor meets the patient. The term makes a statement about the quality of time spent with the patient (as opposed to the length of time spent with the patient) because the patient has had what s/he needs and has been met by the doctor more than half way. This is partly about the patient feeling nurtured, irrespective of whether they can be cured, irrespective of the doctor's technical skills, and *even* irrespective of the doctor's apparently brusque surface manner, provided that beneath that surface the doctor has 'a heart of gold'.

Some Questions
In the light of the above consider the following prompts as you read through your writing and add further to your narrative.

- Were there any dilemmas in meeting the needs of your patient in your case?
- Were there any examples in your case of human being (doctor) meeting human being (patient)? Can you elaborate on what influenced this?
- Were there any examples where you defaulted to a purely technical response to a human need? Can you elaborate on this?

Again make a note of anything that surprised you in doing this writing, ready for use in Chapter Eight.

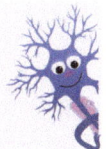

Invisible 6: Seeing the wider perspective around the case TURQUOISE

Figure 2.6.8 The Wider-Perspective Heuristic

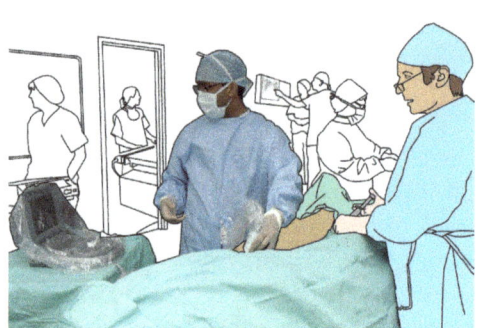 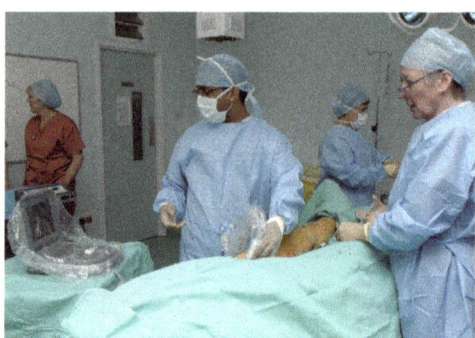

This heuristic shows two pictures of the same scene, but in the picture on the left the background is not highlighted, as the concentration of the surgeons is on the task in hand. They are quite oblivious of what is going on around them. For us too, being very focused on our own practice is particularly important when learning new things and carrying them out for the first few occasions. This is indeed a notable feature in the less experienced.

Increasing expertise, however, 'turns the light' on to what is going on around you, and is depicted in the picture on the right, which shows the background in clear focus. Awareness of the wider context comes with being fluent and capable with the job in hand and therefore being free to be more aware of what is happening beyond you. It is often manifested as increasing confidence and experience and it is what those around you see. Your increased awareness here may be vital in what you are doing.

We first encourage you therefore, to take a step back (metaphorically speaking) and to look through the lens of an interested observer, in order to notice things about the case from a different perspective.

Prompts

- What (if anything) did this Invisible/Heuristic bring to your mind, with respect to your case, about the wider context of medical practice? Make some comment if appropriate. Write in turquoise.
- Was there a wider global perspective to things in your case?
- What did you learn about others involved in this case and your relationship with them?
- Was anything prompted in your mind by this case that normally you just take for granted?
- Did anything surprise you when you were doing this?

> *Again make a note of anything that surprised you in doing this writing, ready for use in Chapter Eight.*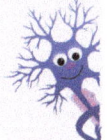

You will now have completed your notes for your first draft of the enriched narrative of your chosen case and the writing will be in a range of colours. Read through the whole account and work on it to ensure that the writing is in separate paragraphs that relate to each of the black bullet points. Try to hear how it sounds and attend to any sentences that do not sound right, making sure they are sentences rather than notes.

This now completes your very first draft. NB: Store this file carefully and use a duplicate of the writing when you are ready to add the next stage. Then you will have evidence of how you built this up. Such evidence may be useful for a variety of purposes, for example, when you are teaching others this whole process.

Refining Your First Draft

The first draft that you have worked on is worthy of refinement. A well-crafted piece of writing is always a joy and brings a sense of great achievement to the writer and makes things clearer both for the writer and the reader. We offer below therefore some ideas you may well follow to refine your first draft.

Your overall aim is to create a clear, precise but vivid narrative that you are proud of and which reflects the efforts that you have put into its creation. It must be honest (without being confessional!) accurate, and measured. Its neatness and readability are important even if it is a piece for exploration and critique only by you yourself. Above all don't *say* how expert you have been but rather *show the evidence* for this, and let the reader decide from that what your level of expertise is. Readers, especially those who know you, will quickly know whether or not you have a realistic view of your abilities.

Writing is a means of learning by helping you recognise your subconscious understanding of events and gives a pleasure of its own to the writer. You may be surprised about your growing desire to write as you find your voice and gain trust and faith in your own ability (Bolton and Delderfield, 2018).

When you have completed your first read through (which should only take a few minutes), give your text a title which captures the importance of this case for you. Remember that the story is substantially about you and needs to be both descriptive and revealing of your thoughts at the time as well as your attitude to your subject. It might help to imagine a trusted colleague sitting at your shoulder as you write and asking yourself what details they need to know to understand your role in the case.

You are now ready to address the following questions.

In creating a good narrative account of the patient case as seen and experienced from your personal perspective as a doctor, use the following list as prompts to sharpen your writing further and to render it immediately vivid and understandable by someone who was not there at the time.

You should ensure that you have:

- written in the first person singular about your own experiences and your personal perspectives on the patient case
- written about *your own* actions in the case, not someone else's
- revealed your own thoughts and emotions where these were significant in the case (whether or not you shared them with the patient)
- identified the influence of your interpretation of the context on your later thoughts and actions
- pinpointed and considered what you previously may have taken for granted.

Reflective writing needs to be vivid and enable the reader to 'be there'. You should also check whether the following about your narrative is true.

- It is about concrete situations and 'is in the moment' (thus helping the writer and the reader to see it or review it vividly).
- It attends in detail to the context of the action/event being reflected on.
- It seeks to study an event/action more deeply and to unpack the thinking and knowing beneath its surface.
- It is narrative in style.
- It sometimes uses figurative language (rich descriptions based on, for example, comparisons using similes and metaphors).

Attend to the above list in the way that suits *you* best and is characteristic of you. Be yourself. Don't strain after ways of writing that you are not comfortable with.

Who is the text for and who is it about?

On your first attempt, you should write the piece just for yourself. This will take away any anxiety that you may have about what another will think. However, in all writing you should consider the following carefully. Whilst there is no golden rule that makes a piece of writing 'right or wrong' it does certainly need to be *appropriate* for the person(s) reading it and the purpose for which you are writing it. In principle therefore, the audience (readership) of the piece is important to consider, as is the purpose of what you are writing and the context in which it will be read. Is it just for you? Is it for your appraiser? Is it to share with learners? Is it to share with patients, managers, the public? What are you trying to achieve through this writing? In what context do you expect the writing to be read?

You may not be aware of it, but you do not really use the same intonation and vocabulary when addressing different people for different purposes in a specific context, whether for an oral interaction or a written one. Think about the differences in vocabulary and tone — that is 'the voice' you would use — between answering questions in a formal interview and rebuking a young child in a domestic situation.

Attending to the voice of your text

The following is offered to help you refine the words you have already written. The principles of what is presented would pertain to any well-written piece. The relationship between writer, subject and audience is what shapes writing. The voice of your text is the personal sound of how you communicate with your reader, which in turn affects how the reader sees you and your subject. The following are the key things that give an individual voice to your writing, and give it authenticity:

- **tone** (the way the words come over because of what you emphasise and your attitude to what you are talking about)
- **style** (the shape and length and the level of formality of the sentence you used and the specific nuance of the vocabulary that you choose)
- **form** (the overall way you structure, shape and order what you have to say).

When you have 'tweaked' your piece of writing, read it aloud again (or better, get someone to read it to you and notice and correct any awkward sentence they stumble over. This is an important refinement whether you are keeping it for your own personal records or preparing it for some other presentation. Store it safely, and make a duplicate version of it to use for the next stage, so that you have evidence of how you built up this writing.

Once captured and worked over to your satisfaction, written reflection, placed on record, has one further potential use. In collecting and presenting several *dated* pieces of reflective writing, each associated with a particular period of time (for example, an attachment for learners, or a year for appraisees), it becomes possible to identify quite quickly some important patterns or pinpoint recurring problems. These will include developments in skill, knowledge, understanding and insight, both about our clinical expertise and ourselves as professionals. This is remarkably easy and does not require more than 3 or 4 pieces to demonstrate such capacities.

Looking from a reader's viewpoint: appreciating the written narrative

Another way of helping you to become clear about how your narrative should be looking, is to offer an example. We do this in the box on page 95. This piece was written by a consultant surgeon learning this process.

We do not offer this for you to give it a 'mark'. Your purpose for reading this is to appreciate the qualities of this sort of writing and to notice its key characteristics or features, in terms of what it tells you about the doctor and how this is achieved. For example, you are bound to deduce some important things about this writer as a doctor that go quite a way beyond what she says about herself, and these are rather more persuasive and believable than if she had stated them as bold facts.

You might think that some of the colours here do not represent the category that you would have put this writing in. We agree that there can be some ambiguity about this. But what really matters here is that the prompts have elicited some important points about the case, that otherwise would have lain dormant, and this will have enriched the account.

Questions to consider as you read each piece
The bolded questions are the key ones, the others are prompts to help you think further.

What are your first impressions about the doctor who has written this case?
- Is there a real person here?
- What gives the writing its 'credibility'?
- Does the writing make you want to read to the end?
- How has this been achieved?

What are the writer's key values and priorities (what does the writer 'stand for')?
- What does the writer say overtly about themselves?
- What can reasonably be deduced about them?
- How would you describe the writer's voice and attitude to their subject?
- How do we learn about 'the person the writer is'?
- Is what the writer says confirmed or contradicted by the way that they say it?

What gives the piece its structure and how does that help the reader to understand what is being said?
- How helpful, to the writer and to the reader, in understanding the case, are the original bullet points?
- How are those bullet points now being used in the main piece?
- How are you helped as reader to find your way through the writing?
- What do the colours highlight about the doctor and the case?
- In what order do you meet the information? (Chronological or not?)
- How clearly is the writing set out, and how well does it flow?
- Is it technically accurate, linguistically? Why does this matter?

How does the author meet and take account of the reader?
- Does the writer overtly acknowledge and take account of the reader and their needs?
- What are the key means of doing this?

- By what means does the writer make the case vivid for the reader?
- How do you know that this is the doctor's personal voice?
- What further information / comment would you like to have been offered?
- What do you discern as a fellow professional about the needs of this writer?

An example of Rainbow Writing by a consultant surgeon

A 49-year-old female librarian was referred to me because of a persistent discharge from her left ear. The history that I elicited from the patient was that she had no hearing in her right ear since birth and had recent problems with persistent discharge from her left ear.

Clinical examination revealed granulomatous disease in a tympanic membrane retraction pocket on the left side. There was no ear canal present on the right side. I sensed her anxiety and reassured her that I would do my best to relieve her problem. I explained that this would involve investigations and the possibility of an operation. I explained my suspicions to her and suggested that the next step would be to order a CT scan.

The patient was referred for a CT scan and the report indicated the presence of cholesteatoma. I reviewed the scan for myself before seeing the patient in clinic.

At the clinic following the scan, I explained to the patient the findings of the scan; namely disease in the left ear (which had poor levels of hearing), but was the patient's only hearing ear. I also explained about cholesteatomatous disease, and the possible outcome, over time, if the disease was left. I gave her the opportunity of asking any questions.

I then discussed the operation for this disease and the risks associated with the surgery (operating on the left ear could leave the patient totally deaf). The complications from surgery are very similar to the risks of leaving the disease but that by operating I hoped to minimise the risk of a complication occurring. She appeared unphased by this idea and showed some relief that something could be done. I was concerned however that she had not understood the possibility of complications.

She was anxious to go ahead with surgery, despite the risk of ending up totally deaf and appeared more concerned about getting back to work than she was about the consequences of a sudden operative complication occurring. Despite hearing complications / risks of surgery she just wanted to get on with the operation and was resigned to the fact that complications occur. Given the patient's reaction, I assumed she had not appreciated what impact a surgical complication would have, in particular the impact that total loss of hearing would have on her life. I had provided the patient with detailed information and believed that she would have been unable to process all this information immediately. I was concerned that once the patient heard about the risk of meningitis / brain abscess (which can occur, though rarely, with this condition) she had focused on this and was not giving any consideration to the other possible complications. I also explained that one of the relative contraindications to surgery on the ear is operating on the patient's 'only hearing ear'. I explained to the patient that though I accepted her expressed desire to have surgery, that I, as her surgeon, wished to ensure that I had reviewed / considered all aspects of her complicated case before proceeding. I explained that I therefore wanted to discuss her case with my colleagues. Initially the patient seemed to be very much of the opinion that I 'knew best', but I was not so convinced. I had a limited experience as a relatively new consultant. I recognised that different surgeons would hold different opinions about whether to proceed with surgery on the left ear or not. I was concerned that my gut instinct, to operate on the patient's left ear, may not have been the opinion held by more experienced surgeons, and I wished to discuss the case with them, to reassure myself that I was doing the right thing for this patient. I had also seen the patient in the middle of a busy clinic, which had been delayed due to an earlier emergency, and was concerned that perhaps circumstances had influenced how I had imparted the information to her. Perhaps the subconscious pressure of needing to finish clinic before the afternoon consultant arrived or just a lack of clarity of thought from a time-pressured clinic had influenced how I had expressed myself on that day. I also wanted to ensure that the patient had fully considered the gravity of the situation. Before she left, I gave the patient an information leaflet about the ear disease, the surgery for this condition and its associated risks. I assumed the patient was concerned enough about her condition that she would read the information leaflet and I hoped that would clarify any issues I had not fully addressed. That way I could have a more informed discussion with the patient at her next outpatient appointment.

Though not entirey unheard of, this was the first time, as a consultant I had come across this type of case (cholesteatomatous disease in an only hearing ear). I also believed that the patient would accept 'the facts' as presented by me and would go with any decision I made. I was concerned that my initial thought (to operate on the left ear, in an attempt to preserve the patient's remaining hearing) might not have been the general consensus opinion held amongst a group of surgeons. I was anxious to do the best by my patient. I was also aware that in the event of a complication occurring and a medico-legal case arising, I wished to be certain that my decision to operate would be considered the most appropriate management for that patient. I wished to be certain that I was doing 'what was right' both for my patient and for myself (a new consultant who had a reputation to build).

I discussed with one of my colleagues about proceeding with surgery on the left ear, and with another colleague about what options were available for the patient if she did go deaf in the left ear after surgery. He first informed me he too would proceed with surgery in the left ear first, but stated that he was not sure if other ENT colleagues elsewhere would do the same. I discussed with another colleague, in another hospital, about what options for hearing rehabilitation were available for the patient if she did go deaf in the left ear after surgery. I was still concerned the patient did not have a realistic grasp of what being totally deaf would be like. I was anxious to explore, prior to proceeding with surgery, future options of providing a hearing aid (in the form of a specialist implanted hearing aid) to the patient, should the need arise. Having discussed this case with two of my colleagues, I felt confident that proceeding with surgery was the correct clinical decision in this patient's case. I also felt reassured that I had considered and explored all appropriate options when making this professional decision. I wonder how I would have felt about operating had I found out that post-operative hearing rehabilitation would not be available / appropriate for this patient.

I then met the patient again in outpatients' department. We had a detailed discussion and I felt, on this occasion, that the patient had in fact considered her options in detail. I made the decision to proceed with the operation, in keeping with the patient's wishes.

During the operation on the left ear I removed the disease from most of the middle ear cavity but was left with the dilemma about removing the pocket over the stapes (the third hearing bone). I left the pocket undisturbed. Removal of this pocket greatly increased the risk to the patient's hearing. Not removing it potentially increased the risk of recurrence of the disease. I left the pocket undisturbed. I did not wish to unduly increase the risk to the patient's hearing. My decision not to operate on that part of the ear was, in my opinion, a considered one. I based my decision partly on my sense of duty to my patient not to put her at undue risk, as there was no disease in that part of the ear at the time of surgery. I also believed that despite our discussions prior to surgery, neither the patient nor I could truly appreciate what impact it would have on her life if the patient were to be rendered totally deaf at the age of 49yrs. I thought that I would find that an extremely difficult situation and assumed finding herself totally deaf all of a sudden would have a similar impact on my patient also.

One month post-operatively, the patient is recovering well from her surgery.

Now go back to your own writing and review it one more time.

Endnote

You are now ready to move to Chapter Seven which will take you through the process of exploring your Clinical Thinking.

> *In summary, Aneumi says: Work over your story so that you tell it in a voice that is alive, personal, and open, in a style that is narrative, in words that are appropriately vivid and in a tone that is professional, friendly and yet intrigued / interested / surprised.*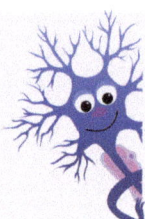

Chapter Seven

Interrogating your Case Narrative to explore your Clinical Decision Making and Professional Judgement

Introduction
A *review* of your current narrative
Exploring your Professional Judgements and Clinical Decision Making
Assessing the quality of your Clinical Thinking
An Example of identifying Professional Judgements and Clinical Decisions
Endnote

Introduction

The purpose of this chapter is to help you interrogate your enriched Case Narrative so that you can come ultimately to a view of the quality of your medical practice in this case (which you will then summarise with the guidance of Chapter 8). From the narrative you have already created, you will first produce an overview of what you have come to understand better, or even for the first time, about your practice. You will then be helped to use the Exploratory Invisibles to spot your professional judgements and then unearth your (often tacit) clinical thinking (the 'working out' underpinning your actions). Then you will be called upon to appreciation the quality of your professional judgements (decision for action) made in this case.

The chronological order of these actions in practice is first clinical thinking and then a professional judgement leading to action. However, because doctors on the whole rarely make their 'workings out' explicit we have chosen, for the purpose of the interrogation of your narrative, to help you first pinpoint your professional judgements and then work back to unpack the tacit decision making underpinning them. Recognising the importance of articulating our clinical thinking that leads to our judgements is a very significant principle for developing professional practice.

This chapter will then end with some help in assessing overall the quality of your clinical expertise in this case, followed by an example of how to present all this.

A review of your current narrative

This is about the content of your writing (as opposed to the construction of it, which you have just attended to). This review will help you consider: the clinical authenticity of the account (its clinical accuracy); the insights gleaned as you engaged in the process of writing (which you have already made a separate note of during the writing and can now record here); and the insights that now come from looking at the account as a whole, and noticing the patterns of colour and the ways you have chosen to describe various elements. The following prompts should help you. As usual, not all may be relevant in every case.

The clinical authenticity
- In retrospect, is the clinical reporting of this case accurate?
- Is the order of events clinically correct?
- Has anything clinically important been omitted?

The insights gained during the process of writing the narrative
- State briefly the new understandings and any surprises you made a note of as you engaged in the process.

An overview of the narrative
Looking now at the account as a whole, write briefly about the following.

- What does the overall pattern of colour so far tell you or suggest, and how does this relate to what you would have expected (eg: what role did medical factual knowledge (seen in red here) actually play in this case and is that what you expect in patient cases? What do other colours throw up as interesting?)
- What now strikes you about the nuance of the words you have used across the piece (eg: is your tone neutral or does it indicate a particular attitude to any aspect of the case?)
- What have you learnt about yourself by *reading this piece*?
- What questions are you left with (if any) at this point?

Exploring your Professional Judgements and Clinical Decision Making

Our Clinical Thinking Pathway (Figure 2.7.1) contextualises the professional judgements made by the doctor during a clinical case. It demonstrates that Professional Judgements shown as the purple tube running throughout the case and, leading to an action for the patient, and a final product professional judgement at the end. The model shows the key influences affecting the doctor's decisions, and probably the patient's too, throughout the whole doctor-patient relationship.

The following pages offer prompts to guide you to identify the elements of your Clinical Thinking.

Figure 2.7.1 The Clinical Thinking Pathway (CTP) and the Influences during treatment

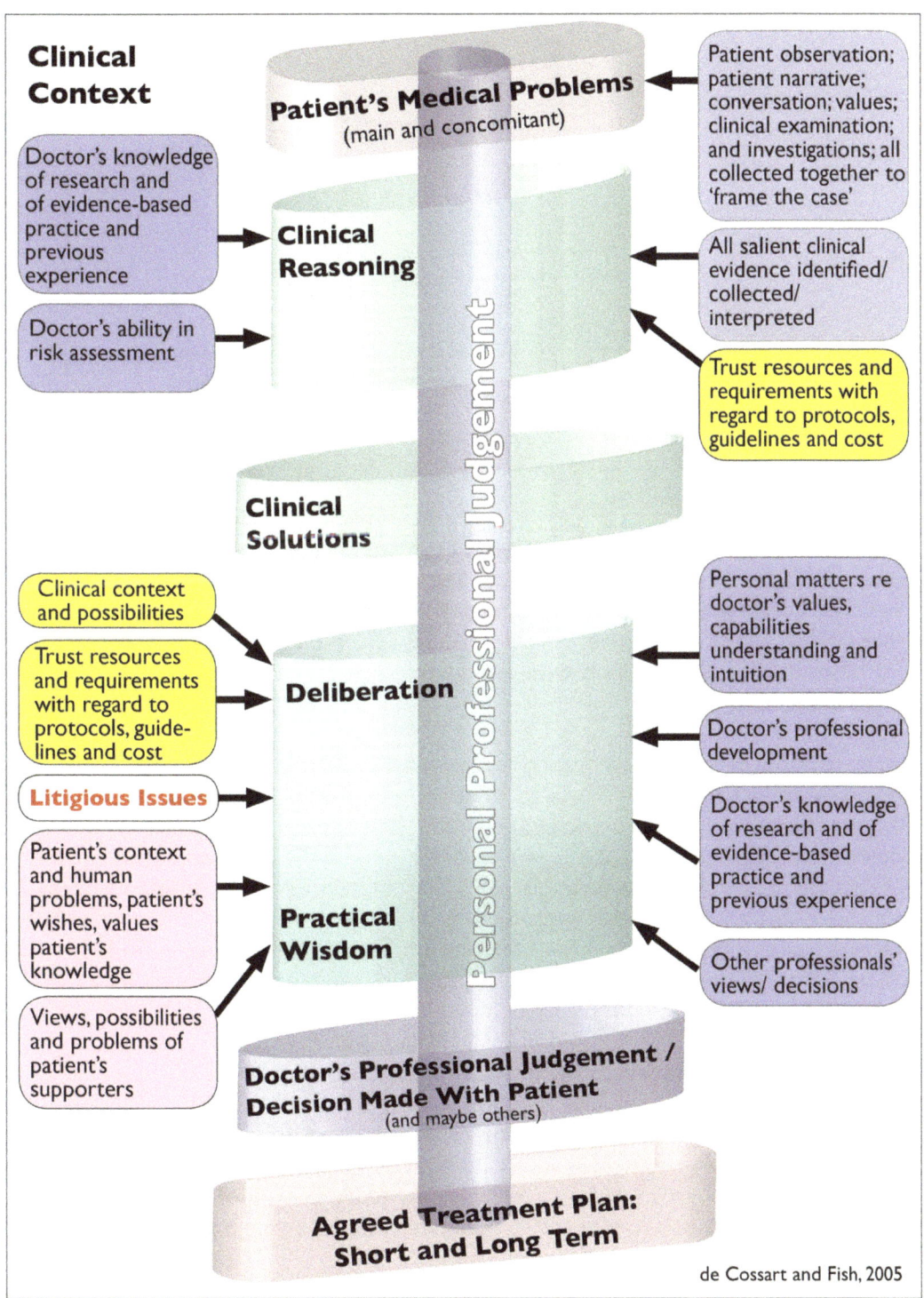

Invisible Seven: Identifying your Professional Judgement **BROWN**

Figure 2.7.2 The Professional Judgement Heuristic

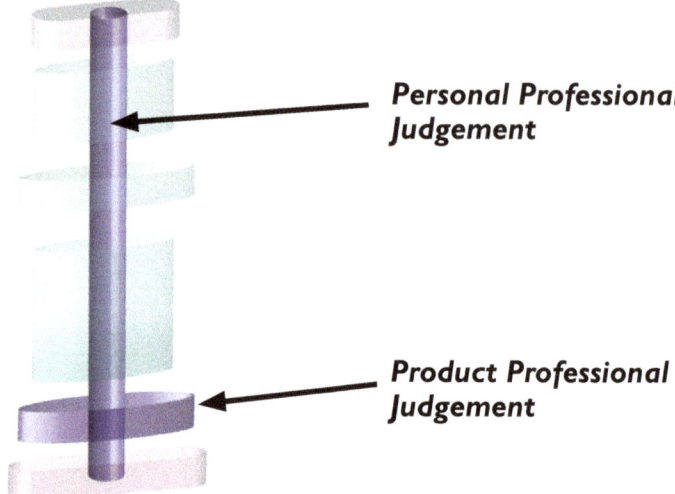

The Professional Judgement Heuristic is shown in Figure 2.7.2 and the two types of professional judgement made in a clinical case are represented in purple. We have come to call the tube running throughout the case 'personal professional judgements'. These tend to be quick decisions often binary in nature, for example: *Should I do another blood test? Should I order another CT scan? Should I call the boss?* The ovoid towards the end of the CTP and leading to wise action, we have called the product professional judgement.

It is quite important to remember that judgements made early in a case will significantly affect the patient's care and will have an influence on the product professional judgement. Without thoughtful consideration, the quality of personal professional judgements, occurring throughout the process, may be overlooked if the product judgement seems satisfactory. It is important that this does not happen or valuable learning may be lost about understanding your tacit drivers. This has a particular importance when teaching supervisees. It is the quality of your judgements throughout your career that will become recognised by others as characterising your unique identity as a medical practitioner.

Identifying Professional Judgements in your narrative

We suggest that in the colour brown you place the words professional judgement and a number to indicate chronology in your text, and follow it with the words Personal Professional Judgement or Product Professional Judgement. Remember to note any surprises that you have experienced in doing this. The following may help you here.

Your Personal Professional Judgements

There will be many more of these. Read through your narrative and at every point that led to an action write in (in brown) 'Professional Judgement'. Give a number in order and indicate that it is a Personal Professional Judgement.

Your Product Professional Judgement

This will be the professional judgement that led to the main treatment plan for the patient eg: to operate on the patient or not, or to advise the beginning of chemotherapy or not.

These will usually occur as the culmination of the whole clinical thinking pathway process, but in a long or complex case there maybe a series, each the culmination of a whole review process of the clinical thinking involved in the patient care. Write into your text, Product Professional Judgement.

Transformative Reflection for Practicing Physicians and Surgeons

Invisible Eight: Exploring your Clinical Decision Making   PURPLE

Figure 2.7.3 The Clinical Decision making Heuristic

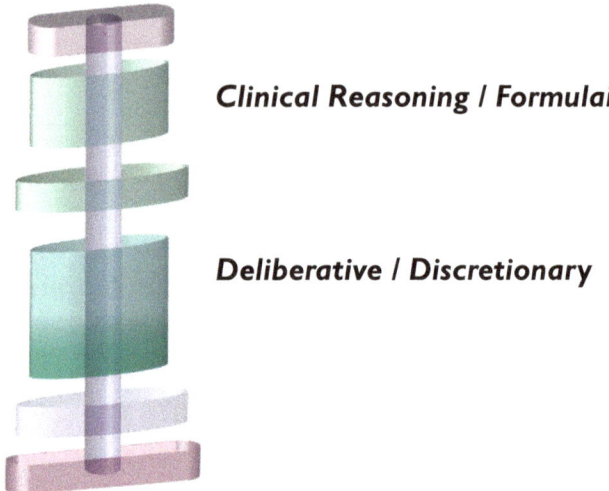

Invisible Eight offers a heuristic for the two forms of clinical decision making that we have described previously: clinical reasoning and deliberation. These are shown on the diagram as different shades of green. The model shows that both types of decision making will happen within every case. The more demanding is deliberative thinking. The quality and consistency of deliberative thinking is a mark of wisdom.

'Clinical Reasoning' in paler green and labelled formulaic at the top end of the pathway is a rather scientific and protocolic process that is a fundamental element of all clinical encounters: that of taking a history, examining the patient, and sending for tests. It is a technical process, requiring technical competence from the practitioner. It leads to a clinical solution about what is wrong with the patient and therefore what — in general — could be the right thing to do for any patient and which everyone would agree. In its simplest and purest form, clinical reasoning construes the complex clinical problem as a technical one and the patient is not focused on as an individual.

By contrast, the bottom half of the Heuristic has varying shades of green becoming darker towards the bottom and labelled 'deliberation'. Deliberation demands from the doctor a more complex thinking process and a humanistic approach to the patient from the doctor and requires them to tailor care to them specifically. It involves the weighing up of (sometimes) competing priorities for which there is no absolute right answer but only what seems at this time best for this specific patient's needs. Deliberation draws on the artistry of the practitioner, requiring them to recognise the unique nature of the situation, to engage in a dialogue with that situation, and to be ready to go beyond the rules (Schön, 1987b: 22). It is based on pragmatic and practical reasoning in which human and equally competing priorities vie for attention, in an order that has to arise from the particulars of the problem and that will therefore be different for different patients. It thus eschews rigid formulae for thinking, using instead an investigative approach to unearthing all the pertinent elements and a reflective and critical approach to prioritising and weighing them up.

Identifying the Clinical Decision making in your narrative

Prompted by the professional judgements you have identified in your case and listed above, ask yourself 'what were my underlying clinical decisions for each of these judgements?' Was my underpinning clinical decision making:

a) **Clinical reasoning** (using the standard formulaic approach, seeking the right thing to do in general). What did you weigh up here?

b) **Deliberative thinking** (using judgements to weigh up competing demands, and seek the best way forward)?

See Figure 2.7.5 as an example

Assessing the quality of your Clinical Thinking

'Arriving at sound professional judgements in complex clinical situations is a key and unavoidable responsibility of the professional' (de Cossart and Fish, 2005). Clinicians are expected by the public to use their specific medical knowledge and skills as well as the qualities of their personhood that they bring to a case. We have written about this previously (Fish and de Cossart, 2007) and have continued to find it resonates with our colleagues in active clinical practice.

Table 2.7.4 provides you with a means of recognising the quality of both forms of judgements. Here, every column offers an important commentary on the judgement and what has led up to it. Again, this can only be used in relation to a given case, and the best evidence of progress will, of course, come from a pattern across cases (taking account of complexity of case and level and stage of career).

Readers are invited to use this table to explore and discuss the quality of their judgements and, for the sake of patients, to raise their aspirations in respect of them, even if the ultimate attainment of wise judgements seems a long way off!

Figure 2.7.4 Some explanation of the quality of the different forms of Professional Judgement

Kind of professional judgement (leading to:)	Response to patient case	Motivation (where the doctor places self in relation to managing the patient)	Questions learner asked themselves
Wise Judgement (enlightenment growing)	Sees each case as needing to be enquired into beyond the obvious, defines what is needed for the best for the patient, can do / obtain what is needed, (checks with senior as appropriate), then does it. Can make rational sense out of intuitive judgement and use pathway both ways up Treats all judgements as potentially provisional and requiring revisiting	Willing and able to put patient's interests first at all times in decision making, even if this risks own interests and position in some way	How can I achieve what is best for the patient? What else should be deliberated upon? Who else should I talk to beyond the obvious team?
Maturing Judgement (developing insight)	Open minded to the complexity of each case; builds on experience. Has a proper respect for conservative management but beginning to balance safety of patient with carefully judged risks	Beginning to put patient first in decision making but still lacks experience to step outside own needs in favour of patient's interests. Beginning to see that you can play it too safe	What should I take into account here? Should I discuss this with my senior?
Self-interested Judgement (need for considerable developmental work)	Selects tactics known to please; closed minded about choices. Chooses what fits limited experience rather than seeing the wider context	Choice of decisions and resultant behaviour designed to enhance own performance and achievements in eyes of consultant	What would my seniors do and how can I please them? What am I personally able do in this case, and how will I do that?
Hasty / Habitual Judgement (recognition that this is unsatisfactory)	Knee jerk reaction / Going through the motions unthinkingly.	Has not even considered that choices are available.	None I've seen this before, haven't I? Why shouldn't I do the same again?

The first column here shows that a hasty or unquestioned habitual judgement (below the red line) will place the doctor in a discrete category of 'unsatisfactory' (which must be retrieved before real development can occur). All other judgements that have been arrived at through some intelligent and conscious thinking, offer promise of progress on a developmental continuum that rises from self-interested decisions to wise judgements. Wise judgement is clearly the aim, but even the most senior doctors may begin the process of formulating a judgement by starting with self-interest, which they then override for reasons we shall see below.

The second column offers in more detail the motivations that lie behind these judgements. It shows that the unsatisfactory judgement is made when the doctor is not motivated to weigh up the complexity of choices available, but merely 'goes through the motions' of being a doctor. The developing doctor, on the other hand, is seen moving through a continuum from concern only for own self-interest, to a real understanding of what is involved in putting the patient first. That is, the doctor moves from concern only with self and the impression made by good performance; through a stage where it begins to be clearer what is involved in putting the patient first, while still clinging conservatively to the preservation of self-esteem; and finally reaches an understanding that genuinely valuing the patient involves transcending all concern for self.

Wise judgement, then, which is something to aspire to, involves balancing reason and emotion in sensing what is best for the patient, gaining a disinterested (detached) interest in the patient, standing up for whatever is best for the patient, and taking a temperate course that is aimed first and foremost at the conquest of the patient's suffering. There is no room here for the arrogant voices of self-preservation, self-concern, self-interest: only for genuine humility, which as T.S. Eliot points out: 'is endless', and which should not be confused with unctuous claims about being 'humble'.

Column three then offers the response to the patient that these motivations result in, and column four offers the doctor examples of the kinds of questions they might ask themselves, (or as teachers, their learners), at points along this continuum.

An Example of identifying Professional Judgements and Clinical Decisions

The example of the consultant's narrative draft you have seen in the previous chapters is shown below with the points of professional judgement (in brown) and type of clinical decision making (in purple) pinpointed in the text. See Figure 2.7.5. Figure 2.7.6 shows how the consultant expanded her underpinning thinking to the professional judgement that she made and Figure 2.7.7 categorises the type of clinical thinking that she believes that she used.

Figure 2.7.5 Pinpointing Professional Judgements and Clinical Decisions

A 49-year-old female librarian was referred to me because of a persistent discharge from her left ear. The history that I elicited from the patient was that she had no hearing in her right ear since birth and had recent problems with persistent discharge from her left ear.

Clinical examination revealed granulomatous disease in a tympanic membrane retraction pocket on the left side. There was no ear canal present on the right side. I sensed her anxiety and reassured her that I would do my best to relieve her problem. I explained that this would involve investigations and the possibility of an operation. I explained my suspicions to her and suggested that the next step would be to order a CT scan. **Clinical Reasoning (1)**, **Professional Judgement (1)**: personal professional judgement. Not all surgeons scan these patients pre-op.

The patient was referred for a CT scan and the report indicated the presence of cholesteatoma. I reviewed the scan for myself before seeing the patient in clinic.

At the clinic following the scan, I explained to the patient the findings of the scan; namely disease in the left ear (which had poor levels of hearing), but was the patient's only hearing ear. I also explained about cholesteatomatous disease, and the possible outcome, over time, if the disease was left. I gave her the opportunity of asking any questions. **Clinical Reasoning (2).**

I then discussed the operation for this disease and the risks associated with the surgery (operating on the left ear could leave the patient totally deaf). **Clinical Reasoning (3)**. The complications from surgery are very similar to the risks of leaving the disease but by operating I hoped to minimise the risk of a complication occurring. **Clinical Reasoning (4) / Deliberation (1)**. She appeared unphased by this idea and showed some relief that something could be done. I was concerned however that she had not understood the possibility of complications.

She was anxious to go ahead with surgery, despite the risk of ending up totally deaf and appeared more concerned about getting back to work than she was about the consequences of a sudden operative complication occurring. Despite hearing complications / risks of surgery she just wanted to get on with the operation and was resigned to the fact that complications occur. Given the patient's reaction, I assumed she had not appreciated what impact a surgical complication would have, in particular the impact that a total loss of hearing would have on her life. I had provided the patient with detailed information and believed that she would have been unable to process all this information immediately. I was concerned that once the patient heard about the risk of meningitis / brain abscess (which can occur, though rarely, with this condition) she had focused on this and was not giving any consideration to the other possible complications.

I also explained that one of the relative contraindications to surgery on the ear is operating on the patient's 'only hearing ear'. **Clinical Reasoning (5)**. I explained to the patient that though I accepted her expressed desire to have surgery, that I, as her surgeon, wished to ensure that I had reviewed / considered all aspects of her complicated case before proceeding. **Deliberation (3)**. I explained that I therefore wanted to discuss her case with my colleagues. **Professional Judgement (2)**: I thought I had made a wise professional judgement here, but could it be interpreted as self-interested professional judgement? Initially the patient seemed to be very much of the opinion that I 'knew best', but I was not so convinced. I had a limited experience as a relatively new consultant. I recognised that different surgeons would hold different opinions about whether to proceed with surgery on the left ear or not. I was concerned that my gut instinct, to operate on the patient's left ear, may not have been the opinion held by more experienced surgeons, and I wished to discuss the case with them, to reassure myself that I was doing the right thing for this patient. I had also seen the patient in the middle of a busy clinic, which had been delayed due to an earlier emergency, and was concerned that perhaps circumstances had influenced how I had imparted the information to her. Perhaps the subconscious pressure of needing to finish clinic before the afternoon consultant arrived or just a lack of clarity of thought from a time-pressured clinic had influenced how I had expressed myself on that-day. I also wanted to ensure that the patient had fully considered the gravity of the situation. Before she left, I gave the patient an information leaflet about the ear disease, the surgery for this condition and its associated risks. **Deliberation (4)**. I assumed the patient was concerned enough about her condition that she would read the information leaflet and I hoped that would clarify any issues I had not fully addressed. That way I could have a more informed discussion with the patient at her next outpatient appointment. **Professional Judgement (3)**: Again was there an element of self-interest here? Or was it a wise judgement to give the patient the leaflet?

Though not entirely unheard of, this was the first time I had come across this type of case (cholesteatomatous disease in an only hearing ear) as a consultant. I also believed that the patient would accept 'the facts' as presented by me and would go with any decision I made. I was concerned that my initial thought (to operate on the left ear, in an attempt to preserve the patient's remaining hearing) might not have been the general consensus opinion held. **Deliberation (5)**. I was anxious to do the best by my patient. I was also aware that in the event of a complication occurring and a medico-legal case arising, I wished to be certain that my decision to operate would be considered the most appropriate management for that patient. I wished to be certain that I was doing 'what was right' both for my patient and for myself (a relatively junior consultant who had a reputation to build.

I discussed with one of my colleagues about proceeding with surgery on the left ear, **Deliberation (6).** and with another colleague about what options were available for the patient if she did go deaf in the left ear after surgery. The first informed me he too would proceed with surgery in the left ear first, but stated that he was not sure if other ENT colleagues elsewhere would do the same. I discussed with another colleague, in another hospital, about what options for hearing rehabilitation were available for the patient if she did go deaf in the left ear after surgery. I was still concerned the patient did not have a realistic grasp of what being totally deaf would be like. I was anxious to explore, prior to proceeding with surgery, future options of providing a hearing aid (in the form of a specialist implanted hearing aid) to the patient, should the need arise. Having discussed this case with two of my colleagues, I felt confident that proceeding with surgery was the correct clinical decision in this patient's case. I also felt reassured that I had considered and explored all appropriate options when making this professional decision. I wonder how I would have felt about operating had I found out that post-operative hearing rehabilitation would not be available / appropriate for this patient. **Professional Judgement (4)**: Maturing / Wise judgement.

I then met the patient again in the outpatients' department. We had a detailed discussion and I felt, on this the, that the patient had in fact considered her options in detail. I made the decision to proceed with the operation, in keeping with the patient's wishes. **Professional Judgement (5)**: wise judgement.

During the operation on the left ear I removed the disease from most of the middle ear cavity but was left with the dilemma about removing the pocket over the stapes (the third hearing bone). I left the pocket undisturbed. Removal of this pocket greatly increased the risk to the patient's hearing. Not removing it potentially increased the risk of recurrence of the disease. **Deliberation (9)**. I left the pocket undisturbed. I did not wish to unduly increase the risk to the patient's hearing. My decision not to operate on that part of the ear was, in my opinion, a considered one. I based my decision partly on my sense of duty to my patient not to put her at undue risk, as there was no disease in that part of the ear at the time of surgery. I also believed that despite our discussions prior to surgery, neither the patient nor I could truly appreciate what impact it would have on her life if the patient were to be rendered totally deaf at the age of 49yrs. I thought that I would find that an extremely difficult situation and assumed finding herself totally deaf all of a sudden would have a similar impact on my patient also. **Professional Judgement (6)**: maturing judgement.

One month post-operatively, the patient is recovering well from her surgery.

Figure 2.7.6 The underpinning thinking to the Professional Judgements
The consultant offers further comment on her professional judgements

As the consultant of this patient I knew that this complex case required me to make many professional judgements along the way. My first judgement of this case was where I made a decision to refer my patient for a CT scan prior to deciding on the appropriate management of her condition. (**Professional Judgement 1**) Not every consultant requests CT scans pre-op but my decision to do so was based on the belief that a scan could offer more information regarding the nature/extent of the disease. Given the complexity of this patient's case, I wanted to be sure I knew the full extent of her disease to be able to share this with her and allow it to inform my intended action and thus I felt doing the test was in her best interests.

When I next met with the patient, it was clear she wished to proceed with surgery without further delay. She wanted to get back to work as soon as possible. However, I decided not to agree to her request immediately. I decided to defer my decision on management until I had discussed her case with my colleagues (**Professional Judgement 2**). In this instance it is possible to believe that I was in fact acting out of self-interest, as my choice of decision was designed to enhance my own performance and achievement. I did not want to make the wrong decision. At the time of making my judgement I believed it was because I was aware of the 'lottery' effect and did not want the patient to 'suffer' due to my decision. However, it is clear I also had the worry of medico-legal issues in mind. I was concerned not just that I was making the right decision for this patient, but that I would be seen to have done so by my peers and would be able to defend my decision (to operate on this woman's left ear) to my opponents (those who would not proceed with surgery in this case) if called to do so. My decision in part therefore must be considered to be a self-defensive judgement.

Having made my decision to discuss this patient's case with my colleagues, I proceeded to give my patient an information leaflet on the disease and surgery (**Professional Judgement 3**). This is not something I do for all my patients (as I often fear the information will scare them too much) but on this occasion I deliberately decided to give the patient the information. Again, on reflection, I can question whether this was based on wise judgement (believing that providing this patient with all available information was in her best interests). Perhaps instead it was a self-defensive judgement, allowing me to work through my clinic as efficiently as possible (rather than taking even more time to talk to my patient); while still making me feel like I have done something for my patient?

My decision to discuss with a colleague the options available for hearing rehabilitation (**Professional Judgement 4**) though were done with the patient's best interests at heart (Wise Judgement) and showing perhaps signs of maturing judgement and enlightenment, but it did at the same time, I think, put me at risk of scorn from some colleagues by exposing what might have been seen as a weakness on my part. I believe that I was wise in considering the future options available to my patient but at the time was questioning myself about my reason for doing this. Was I pursuing this in order to reassure myself about what else that could still be done for her, in the event of a complication arising? By exploring this before surgery, I offering my colleague the opportunity to undertake the primary surgery if he felt that was the right thing to do. It therefore appeared that I was considering my patient's interests above all else but, in reality, did I approach this colleague because I needed to be sure, for me, that I was doing all that I could. My decision was therefore not entirely wise maybe even a self-defensive one.

Finally, I did decide to operate on this patient, having satisfied my own and the patient's questions about this case (**Professional Judgement 5**): Wise Judgement. But, as is so often the case, just when it seems an answer has been found another unexpected situation arises. On this occasion, having no further opportunity to engage in collaborative conversation with my patient, I was faced with an unexpected finding during the operation. Intraoperative decision making is part of the role of the surgeon. At the time I felt like my management decision, once again, held the potential for disaster either way. My patient could, if I proceeded to try to remove this pocket of disease entirely, be left deaf immediately after the surgery or she could be left with an area (the pocket) in which disease could reoccur, potentially causing a complication at a later date. I decided to leave the pocket intact to be observed in clinic in the years to come (**Professional Judgement 6**). Once again at the time of surgery I believed that I had made a wise judgement, with the patient's best interests at heart. There was no disease in that area at that time, and operating could have had drastic consequences (leaving the patient totally deaf). Perhaps, on reflection, my decision may have been a little more about playing it safe for me (maturing judgement) than I would at first have admitted?

Figure 2.7.7 The categorisation of the Clinical Thinking
The consultant offers further comment on the clinical thinking underpinning her professional judgements

In my management of this patient, I firstly framed the case by gathering information about the patient's history and by recording my clinical examination findings. Having completed my initial assessment I immediately began my clinical reasoning stating '... my suspicions' and taking the decision to investigate further by referring the patient for a CT scan (**Clinical Reasoning 1**).

I continued my clinical reasoning during that initial consultation by explaining to the patient about this type of ear disease, its natural progression and associated risks, as well as informing her about the management options and surgery. These points were all raised in discussion of the disease and surgery in general (**Clinical Reasoning 2, 3 and 4**) but I immediately found myself considering the impact of the present on this patient who only had one functioning ear (in terms of hearing). I hoped to minimise the risk to the patient by performing surgery but it is clear from my use of language both to the patient and here in my discussion that I was not convinced that that would in fact be the outcome (**Deliberation 1**).

Again I reverted to clinical reasoning and discussion with the patient; discussing the golden rule of ear surgery (never operate on the patient's ear, if it is the only ear they can hear with) (**Clinical Reasoning 5**). I believe my main reason for doing so was firstly so that the patient could have all the facts in order to make her decision regarding her management. I also believe that by having these discussions I was hoping to glean further information about the patient; her values, wishes and perhaps also determine her ability to make a fully informed decision (**Deliberation 2**). I was at this point putting myself at risk of being seen by the patient as perhaps 'unsure' of what I should do. I weighed up that it was better to be in full knowledge of the facts and share with her all the potential risks.

This lead me on to my own deliberation 'as her surgeon' of this 'complicated case' (**Deliberation 3**). Did I have enough experience on which to base my decision regarding this patient's management? What would my colleagues do if faced with the same case? I was anxious that the patient's management was not influenced by the lottery of her seeing me rather than another of my consultant colleagues in outpatient clinic.

I recognised that I can express myself better on some occasions that on others. I pondered the fact that my ability to express myself when under time-pressure in a delayed clinic might have influenced the patient's decision unduly. Had my explanation been clear enough on this occasion so as to allow me to obtain fully informed consent at that time? My deliberation on these issues (**Deliberation 4**) caused me to offer the patient written information regarding her condition, such that she could review this information later. Thus I hoped that when I next met the patient I would be able to have a more detailed and informed collaborative discussion with her.

I deliberated on the medico-legal aspects of the case. If a complication did arise, would I be able to defend my decision to the patient, to myself or in a court of law? Had I taken every possible step to ensure I was offering the best possible care to this patient? (**Deliberation 5**)

In order to ensure that I could defend my decision, I chose to involve other professional colleagues in my deliberation. With one of my colleagues, I discussed whether the patient should have surgery on this left ear at all (**Deliberation 6**). I subsequently discussed with another colleague, based at a different hospital, if the option of rehabilitation would be available to this patient if a complication arose during surgery. I believed that knowing whether an option for hearing rehabilitation was available to my patient could influence her / my decision to proceed (**Deliberation 7**). I also understood that it is often easier to do a second operation on a patient's ear if you have performed the primary surgery. Knowing I could not perform the implant surgery required for rehabilitation, I therefore discussed the option of the implant surgeon performing the primary surgery also (**Deliberation 8**). He felt this was not necessary in this patient's case. I found this supportive and reassuring.

Armed with this information I met with the patient again. Once again we entered the clinical reasoning phase; discussing her understanding of the disease and her wishes regarding her condition (**Clinical Reasoning 6**). With a greater understanding of my patient and her wishes, as well as a greater confidence in my own understanding of the case, I then deliberated further (**Deliberation 9**) and was able to arrive at a (product) professional judgement during that meeting in outpatients.

My decision making did not end there however. During the surgery I was once again faced with a number of unexpected issues. The extent of the disease and the area of the ear involved forced me to consider the option of not operating on / removing all the disease (**Clinical Reasoning 7**). On this occasion I considered the possible outcomes regarding removal / leaving the disease, in light of my knowledge of the patient and her wishes. I weighed this up in the light of my own experience and understanding of how this 'pocket' disease differed from the expected disease (cholesteatoma) (**Deliberation 10**). I made a professional decision to leave this less aggressive disease in situ and to monitor it in the future, thus minimising the risks to this patient at this time.

Endnote

In attempting to make very clear both the elements of clinical thinking and how to explore professional judgement, we have inevitably simplified a number of things. Of these, we have already warned of the dangers of the reductionism that models bring. We now issue a warning about the need to use these processes in more complex ways. We have presented the pathways as leading doctors directly to a clear judgements, but would strongly emphasise the fact that in real practice, clinicians will always go back over the pathway and revisit the decisions and the thinking that led to them. And this is particularly so when elements that do not fit emerge and are faced squarely. This will be so, for example, when the diagnosis at the end of the clinical reasoning pathway is still somewhat uncertain. The first decision being made at this point enables the progression of care of the patient, but is not necessarily the final diagnosis.

We emphasise then that as a general rule, where at any stage uncertainty remains about the accuracy of diagnosis, recycling through the pathway must always be carried out.

We hope that you will agree that several pieces of writing by a doctor over a period of time will not only help them develop their thinking, but also be a testament to their commitment to their own development and their developing insights and wisdom.

Chapter Eight

Summarising the results of your efforts

Introduction
The emergence of key insights and new understandings
Responding to Appraisal and the GMC requirements
Endnote and a caution

Introduction

This chapter offers some guidance on drawing from all you have done so far in order to summarise your key insights and new understandings about yourself, your clinical practice and your emerging ideas for your continuing professional development. Your aim should be to make a logical and succinct summary of what you have learned and how this will influence your further development. The nuance of your summary will depend on how it will be used. Will it be: just for your personal file; for sharing with learners; for your appraisal; for negotiating your continuing professional development? The narrative of your case and your exploration of your clinical thinking is the evidence to support your summary of what you have learned by reflecting on this case from your practice. There is an example at the end of the chapter of a summary written by the consultant surgeon whose work you have been reading about in the previous few chapters.

The emergence of new key insights and understandings

It would be helpful here if you looked back over the various colours in your rainbow draft which are likely to give you clues and evidence for your summary. For example: What is the predominant colour? What is your reaction to that? What was the colour least seen? Are you surprised by this and how will you comment on this?

What did I learn newly about myself as a person and a professional?

The process of reflective writing that we have taken you through will have caused you to see your practice from a different perspective. The questions below aim to help you to summarise your personal insights.

- What does my commitment to doing this (Transformative Reflective Writing) say about my willingness to learn something new?
- Was I surprised by anything that emerged about me as a person? For example: Was I more thoughtful than I had expected? Were there things that made me pleased/ displeased/ annoyed?
- Did anything important arise about me as a professional?
- Is there anything here that I might share with supervisees in a teaching session?

- What new personal insights emerged?
- How will all this influence my future practice, my teaching and my need for professional development?

What did I learn newly about myself as a professional doctor?

The following questions may help you to clarify the quality of your Clinical Reasoning

- How much did I rely on the validity and reliability of information provided by others?
- How did I decide that I had sufficient information to make the decision about a plan of care for the patient?
- How did my own values and humanity enable me to relate to the case?
- What factors did I discount?
- How did I interpret test results? Did I question any of them?
- What did I think of the quality of interpretations being offered by others?
- Did I differentiate between my opinions and my knowledge? How did I recognise or see this in relation to what I would do?
- Did I critique my decision in terms of its appropriateness for this patient? How did I prioritise this case? How did I choose between competing demands? How did I allow for the ambiguities of this particular case?
- How did I listen to my intuitions? Did I discount my own interests? Did I recognise the need for a period for reconsideration of the treatment plan?

Responding to Appraisal and the GMC requirements

You may find you wish to use your writing for your appraisal. We offer the table below to link the four domains in the Appraisal process, required by the GMC, and how each Invisible can help you to use key cases in your practice to provide evidence for each domain.

Table 2.8.1 How the Invisibles help your response to the four GMC Domains (adapted from Fish and de Cossart, 2013, 116)

GMC Domains	Reflective Case Evidence
Knowledge, Skills and Performance	What evidence is there in my reflections on this case, and of my understanding of my knowledge, skills and performance as a doctor? See the following for clues: • context **(Invisible 1)** • my knowledge **(Invisible 4)** • the breadth of skills in general and speciality specific practice **(Invisible 4)** • the quality of my professional judgements and clinical decision making **(Invisibles 7 & 8)** • what underpins my 'performance' as a doctor? **(Invisible 1 to 8)**

GMC Domains	Reflective Case Evidence
Safety and Quality	What evidence is there in this case of my understanding of the need to ensure safety and quality? See: • context **(Invisible 1)** • the quality of my professional judgements and clinical decision making **(Invisibles 7 & 8)** • recognition of the ambiguities and complexities of practice **(Invisibles, 1, 5, 6, 7, 8)**
Communications, Team work and Partnership	What evidence is there in this case of my understanding of and my involvement in Communications, Team work and Partnership? See: • my professionalism **(Invisible 3)** • my relationship with the wider clinical team **(Invisibles 1-8)** • being prepared to use my writing to improve understanding between team members (evidence of what I have shared orally and in writing)
Maintaining Trust	What written evidence of candour is offered in the narrative? Several cases over a period of time will highlight trends and consistency of my capacity as a clinician. What evidence do I offer of my insight into what constitutes my clinical expertise and growing professional identity **(Invisibles 1-8)**

How does this inform and justify your plans for CPD?

All doctors will need to make a case for how their continuing professional development is planned and structured. Using appropriate case narratives to show what you do and how appropriate CPD will support your growth and development, is a powerful means of structuring and providing for your argument.

Responding to complications and complaints

The structure that we have offered through the TRP works extremely well as a framework for unpacking your actions and decision making in cases of complications and complaint. Used by each member of a clinical team in response to contentious cases, the process brings each member's own analysis and insights to case discussions and hugely empowers members to engage in the process and sharpen their thinking.

How did you find the TRP and how will you continue to use it (or not!)?

This question requires honesty. If you have struggled, do not be too hasty to dismiss the process. The first few attempts may be longwinded, but the process will become quicker and more fluent with effort and time. It will become part of everyday practice and thinking rather than just written exercises in private. The figure overleaf offers a summary of the case that you have read in the previous chapters.

Figure 2.8.2 A Summary of one consultant's use of the TRP

I have summarized my key learning points below as a series of bullet points. They are in no particular order of priority but I believe each offers a specific point.

- When I first started Reflective Writing I found it quite time-consuming. However, as I have become more familiar with the process it not only influences how I write but how I think in clinical practice.
- The writing has helped me clarify my thinking and therefore be more confident and articulate in explaining to others my argument for my actions.
- In this case I was surprised how many times I seemed to be exercising with the patient my thoughts on clinical reasoning. It caused me to consider how time-pressures might influence my patience in doing this. My deliberation prior to the surgery about this case helped considerably my need for an 'on the hoof' deliberative decision during the actual operation. This is something I must remember to highlight when teaching young surgeons.
- I was surprised at how many judgements I made and this has sharpened my listening to trainees (and others!) about how they relate their actions and decision making. It has changed how I ask them questions. I now want to them first to explain 'what they think they should do in a particular patient case' (Final step of the Clinical Thinking Pathway), rather than starting at the top end of the Clinical Thinking Pathway (the standard way of offering a case). I now expect my trainees to start their response to me on ward rounds and in clinic when presenting a case, at the end of the clinical thinking pathway, leaving me to tease out of them the clinical reasoning and deliberation they engaged with along that pathway. At first they do not find this easy because it is not what they are used to!
- This piece is a useful teaching resource.
- I believe this piece would be useful as evidence for my appraisal for demonstrating my commitment to: Communications, Partnership and Teamwork and Maintaining Trust.
- I now have experience that this can be educational when as a team activity each member shares their own Rainbow Writing for discussion.

Endnote and a caution

Reflective practice carried out in this way should perhaps contain a health warning. If abused and used badly it could be harmful. It is always best to share your activity with a trusted and wise professional medical colleague. This will enrich your understanding. Never up-load a piece of your reflective writing to any digital platform without sharing it and refining it so that it offers your authentic voice and information you are prepared to share publicly. Remember the main purpose of this exercise is for you to understand yourself better and to plan better the focus of your professional development. In so doing you will be better able to share the complexities of your practice with clinical colleagues, managers, patients and the wider public as appropriate.

Part Three

Preparing for and planning to teach Transformative Reflection

Introduction to Part Three

In Part One, we presented in depth the social and professional contexts and the traditions of Reflective Practice within which we have developed the process of and resources for Transformative Reflection as a new approach to improving medical care.

In Part Two, we offered the details of the hidden influences (which we call 'The Invisibles'), that have shaped how doctors think and work, and have guided our newly refined version of reflection which we have developed within and beyond the previous traditions of Reflective Practice.

We outlined how those resources can be used by medical practitioners to explore in deep detail a patient case. We demonstrate how, having listed in bullet points a case of a patient one has cared for, it is possible, step by step, to use the Invisibles and their prompts to enrich the developing narrative with details of the doctor's or surgeon's actions and thinking processes and to engage in an interrogation of the enriched narrative to uncover the clinical thinking, the deliberations and the professional judgements that underpinned that patient's entire care. We have used a real patient case (duly anonymised) to provide a clear example of every stage of the process.

Here in Part Three, we attend to teaching this process to a range of medical practitioners from the youngest to the most experienced, by using TRP on a chosen case that the individual learning doctor/surgeon has personally managed. Again, we support this process with real examples.

This Part provides two chapters. The first of these offers some new ways of understanding education as a practice in its own right and the resulting and inevitable changes to how teachers conduct themselves and interact with their learners. It also, therefore, indicates how learners might respond. In short, it shows how to attempt to educate in the moral mode of practice, which seeks to develop a rounded human being, rather than simply a technical trainer who focuses on rules and how to obey protocols.

This prepares the way for the second chapter in Part Three, which takes the readers step by step, to engage learners in critically examining and working with TRP. Here we offer: a whole short programme for teaching those meeting The Invisibles for the first time; a plan for teaching a single session within that programme; some advice for developing further those doctors and surgeons who already have some experience of TRP; ways to improve the professional conversations between teacher and learner about reflection; advice on what new learners should read about reflection; and ways of assessing the written results of TRP.

Readers should note that it is courting failure to attempt to teach a process one has not first learnt and critiqued for oneself. We recommend very strongly that before entering into Part Three, readers should attend first to Parts One and Two of this book.

Chapter Nine

Preparing to teach your junior colleague to engage in transformative reflection: educational starting points

Introduction
Understanding how to work in the moral mode of educational practice
Starting with your learner: seeing them anew
The learner and the formal PGME curriculum
New roles for the teacher and learner
Understanding the role of talking and writing for learning
The importance of using assessment to nurture the learner
Endnote

Introduction

Readers are encouraged to use this chapter to explore ways of raising the quality of education offered by supervisors in PGME and particularly the teaching of The Transformative Reflective Process (TRP), because if properly understood it will have a profound effect on the whole of a doctor's lifetime of both teaching and learning and on how doctors present themselves to those they serve. This is not to dispute that a supervisor's first duty is to ensure that the doctors they supervise are safe and capable in their current medical practice.

The structure of the chapter

We begin here with a distilled overview of the educational beliefs of those who think like educators. You are invited to compare them with what you have already understood about the practice of education. This first section will help you to see the basis of a teacher's priorities both in planning and in teaching. For the educator, the learner is the centre of their interest and focus. What the teacher does is entirely designed to serve the educational and human needs of the learner. Those needs are best understood by the educator, who, while taking account of the learner's interests, can see through any of their exuberant but somewhat inappropriate 'wants' to their real educational needs; who knows the learner well in order to make these judgements; and who is best suited, therefore, to guide them through the educational landscape ahead. Getting to know your learner as a person and a doctor as soon as possible, and seeing them anew as whole human beings, are both therefore vital elements in good teaching. This demands of the clinical supervisor some courage to go beyond the formal PGME curriculum which has nothing to say about the person the learner is. The formal curriculum is an essential foundation for supporting learning, but the teacher *in situ* has to tailor this to the learner's individual circumstances and the practical context of their current clinical practice.

This overview is followed by a section that indicates the differing roles for the teacher and the learner according to the different learning events within a programme. This will help you to know how best to use your own time face-to-face alongside the learner, and to focus more sharply the educational requirements and activities of the learner in working alone between those meetings. This deployment of yourself and your learner will also be shaped by your understanding of the roles of talking and of writing in learning, which are discussed next. Finally, you will need to understand a little about assessment as an educational process, and the significant difference between an assessment that provides data in figures for the recorded end result and that which uses words as evidence.

We shall now turn firstly then to an overview of some educational beliefs that we have found well received by and helpful to the many consultants we have taught to teach what we now call Transformative Reflection. What follows will help anyone who teaches professionals in practice to begin to develop the basis of what is involved in 'thinking like a teacher'.

Understanding how to work in the moral mode of educational practice

We see the practice of education, like the practice of medicine, as essentially a moral and intellectual endeavour. That is, it seeks to *serve* individuals and society by providing 'a good' in the moral sense. In medical practice the good aimed at is sound health for individuals and society wherever possible; in education, the good aimed at is improved ability for all to understand and to conduct themselves better. In law it is supposed to be 'justice' for all. Thus education is about a change or transformation that produces improvement for the individual and for society.

All serious *practices* work within or in response to a tradition. Education has a rich tradition that goes back to the Greeks 500 years before the birth of Christ. The conversation across 2,500 years about ideas that should guide worthwhile education have shown training as providing a change in surface behaviour but without necessarily altering our way of seeing the world, whereas education offers individuals and society seriously beneficial changes in being, thinking, understanding, and doing. Here, new understanding that has been internalised, shows on the surface but is about conduct driven by new and more civilised ideas and beliefs. The argument is as follows. (With acknowledgement to Hansen, 2001.)

- Some people want to learn only the skills of teaching and not bother with the underlying thinking. They want the technical aspects only. (Surgery could be like that too, but wouldn't be good practice.) Thus to focus only on the *means* of teaching (the 'how to') is sterile. It then becomes: a job with a task to

transmit knowledge; an occupation where those outside it set the terms and conditions and the activities carried out.
- To focus instead only on what you are trying to achieve in teaching, can lead to 'outcomes-focused' approaches, where the end product is all that matters, this leads to: producing productive members of society, who are successful and compliant workers. This is dangerous and equally un-educational.
- Teaching as a practice has its own integrity — to those who are thoughtful about what they do as teachers.
- Teachers should first determine what they care about [say the qualities of practising doctors they are 'bringing up' and their service to patients and society] and then craft a conception of teaching that coheres with that determination.' (Hansen, 2001: 4)
- Teachers who give their planning and their practice intellectual and moral substance are also echoing the components of teaching that have developed over time.

That is:
- they are intellectually attentive to learners

- they build positively on what learners know, can do, feel and think, with an eye to increasing their knowledge of the world and of how to continue to learn within it

- they are morally attentive to learners by being alert to learners' responses to opportunities to *grow as persons* (to become more rather than less thoughtful about ideas, and more rather than less sensitive to others' views and concerns)

- they are mindful that every learner is unique, with a distinctive set of dispositions, capabilities, understandings and outlooks.

Thus, the bonds between teacher and learner are intellectual and moral, pertaining to their emerging knowledge, understanding and growth as persons, and so the concept *'person'* is central to the practice of teaching. Attending to the learner as a person is thus important, and offering that learner a teacher who is a person as well as a professional, is also important.

All this is what an educator sees as part of *'being* a teacher'.

Teaching in the moral mode of (postgraduate) educational practice

This means three key things:

1. Making explicit for yourself as the teacher:

    - the human and humane as well as the technical aspects of patients' needs

- the human and humane as well as the technical demands of medical practice in all its complexity;
- deducing from this analysis the educational imperatives to be working on with learning doctors.

2. Seeing educational practice as attending to:

- learners 'being and becoming' as persons and professionals
- their thinking, decision making processes and professional judgements
- their learning of knowledge and skills defined in their curriculum.

3. This means recognising that:

- *your being as a doctor and a teacher* will have a profound impact on your learner as an important model for that learner
- you are an advocate for the kind of education necessary for developing a wise doctor. (A wise doctor is one who practises with the best interests of the whole patient at their mind and heart, using their expertise with sound professional judgement to tailor the care they offer to the patient's own unique circumstances).

This is turn means clarifying for oneself:

- what does and does not conduce to engaging in education and medicine in the moral mode of practice
- one's commitment to work to support worthwhile PGME and where necessary to resist the narrowness of the demands made by the curriculum and by the pressure of daily practice, by the expectations of the NHS, government, Royal Colleges, and the media
- one's commitment to educating the wise doctor — if necessary in opposition to any requirements of external agents that are inimical to this.

In summary, *the moral mode of practice in Postgraduate Medical Education* is about aspiring to understand and make explicit for oneself how one sees the practice of medicine, and what kinds of education will conduce to developing a wise doctor. It also demands that one uses this analysis to critique what external agents require and where necessary seeing these as mere basic requirements while seeking to enrich them in additional ways which though not required are not precluded. This is where the courage we mentioned earlier comes in.

Starting with your learner: seeing them anew

One of the foremost characteristics of teaching in the moral mode of practice involves the teacher seeing the learner anew — as an individual who is central to that teacher's thinking.

This is about recognising the need to start — in thinking, planning and teaching — from:

- where the learner is
- who the learner is
- where the learner aspires to be and what they seek to become
- what the learner needs now.

This is likely to lead the teacher to work to facilitate the learner's development as a professional person, a life-long learner and a good clinician who offers safe quality care to patients. Such a teacher considers the importance of developing the learning doctor as a whole person and argues that, since personality, character and spirituality are key elements in being a doctor, PGME teachers should seek to attend educationally to the person their learner brings to both medical practice and to their own education. This will require the teacher to understand the wants as well as the needs of the learner and be rigorous, fair and attentive to ensuring that they are offered educationally sound resources and processes.

Seeing the learner anew as the above suggests, ensures the establishment of a very different educational relationship from that normally found currently in PGME. It creates a more fruitful and enjoyable starting point for teaching, where the learner is seen as a fellow practitioner and a person who has a range of needs and who also brings important contributions to the teaching. This means that the learner should be a key agent in the educational process. This is not, however, at all the same as simplistically 'giving the learner what they say they want' (which is often not related at all to what they need)!

Only by studying the learner can the teacher attend to them as a person. Given this, the educational interaction between them, then inevitably gains a different dynamic from that found in much traditional PGME where it is routinely assumed that there is no time to engage in depth with learners. (We usually find time to spend on what matters to us.) Improved interaction between learner and teacher results from establishing a sound relationship between them, and the learning becomes dialogic such that the time spent together educationally is used more profitably. In current PGME in the UK this tends to evolve only as the learner becomes more senior and experienced.

The paradox here is that the learner's formal curriculum, being technically oriented, does not seriously recognise that attending to the person the learning doctor is should be part of the syllabus. A teacher who has seen the implications of the moral mode of practice, and who has a strong sense of what matters educationally, recognises that the learner's ontological dimensions (the learner's being) as well as their epistemological needs (their theoretical knowing and their skills) must be attended to (in terms of time and resources). This can be attended to either in addition to, or somehow inside, the formal curriculum to which the learner has an entitlement. This means taking a different approach to the curriculum, the Learning Agreement and the arrangements for learning on each clinical attachment. A teacher persuaded of the value of this might also recognise the need to work to influence that formal curriculum nationally and also to argue locally for more time for education. This is an example of what Palmer (1998) means by the courage needed by teachers.

Understanding what a curriculum is and the importance of moral agency

A curriculum is a carefully planned educational programme. It may be a set of rigid requirements to be followed unquestioningly thus depriving the teacher of any educational agency. Or it might be a set of flexible guidelines that rely on the teacher to interpret what should be learnt in each learner's own context. At the level of principle, it is: an attempt to communicate the essential principles and features of an educational proposal in such a form that it is open to critical scrutiny and capable of effective translation into practice. (Stenhouse, 1975: 4.)

Teaching is an intentional activity. Ideas and understanding do not just emerge as you go along in a learning conversation — although one of your intentions should be to capitalise on anything unexpected that does emerge, and you should always be flexible enough to respond to this need while you are together. Thus, it is important, if you are to use your short time together as significantly as possible, to have thought through the whole logic that will guide your educational work. Such a guide is called 'a curriculum'.

A curriculum is not merely a syllabus which lists the topics to be taught and learned. A curriculum is a properly designed plan for an educational programme, but it is not a protocol to be followed thoughtlessly. Indeed, whenever we do something, we have often tacit ideas that inform what and how we act. For a teacher, these ideas spring from underlying assumptions and beliefs about the activities of teaching, learning and assessment. In worthwhile education, these ideas come through an educational philosophy (see Fish and Coles, 2005). It follows that educational practice cannot be properly developed without these matters (the very educational ideas upon which teachers base their practice) being articulated and explored, and that teachers have a moral commitment to the welfare of learners to understand, express, explore and develop their curriculum, just as doctors have a moral imperative to continue to refine and develop the medical care they provide for patients.

A curriculum, which is an educational policy, finds its expression in practice and needs to be developed *from* practice. Thus, a curriculum may be written or rewritten (**designed**) on paper, and refined in practice (**developed**). But these processes are intertwined — that is they develop and refine each other. As a process that is enacted upon the ground of practice it requires negotiation between learners and teachers. Thus any outline curriculum we might offer the reader can only be properly enacted in practice and for that, the teacher should retain the agency of deciding what to do and how.

Our values are what drive our choices here, and we cannot easily be committed to — or act upon — those ideas and processes which are in conflict with our own values. That is why those engaged in teaching must be permitted a major voice in shaping the curriculum they offer, and why teaching involves negotiating with the learner, whose values and beliefs also need to be recognised.

The curriculum is determined as much by what is not offered, what is omitted, and what has been rejected, as it is by positive decisions. Further, we would wish to argue that unless those who design, or who influence the design of a curriculum, base their work on educational *understanding*, many learning opportunities are likely to be unrecognised and lost. With this in mind, it will be possible to critique any postgraduate medical or other curricula.

> **Note:**
>
> Where the teacher's educational agency is concerned, important issues arise as to how far the written curriculum is a guideline or a protocol! It is a learner's legal entitlement. But it is also the teacher's moral responsibility to tailor it to the specific needs of a given learner in their given context, and for the teacher to be true to their own educational values, vision and philosophy.
>
> These are part of the tensions the supervisor has endlessly to deliberate about and to solve. They also have to adjudicate (often on the spot) between the demands of service and the needs of education, both of which are ultimately about safe patient care! This is not a matter of 'either / or', but a matter of emphasis, which will demand the educational judgement of the supervisor, who needs to remember that patient service in all its complexities is the key resource for teaching and learning in the clinical setting and that it should not be seen as separate from educating the supervisee.

The learner and the formal PGME curriculum

As nationally published documents, the formal curricula for PGME (the Foundation, Core and Specialty curricula) have been drawn up by national experts and should (but do not always) contain far more than a syllabus (which merely lists content to be covered). For more details see Fish and Coles, 2005.

In fact, a formal national curriculum can only ever be a basis for the local, active, education of practitioners on the ground. Judgements therefore have to be made by each teacher about what each specific learner needs educationally, and how this relates to what has been published. Thus, the first judgement is about how to regard the learner's curriculum! We add here our disappointment that the ninety-nine curricula on the GMC website are all disparate documents when the ontological and humane elements ought to be (and rarely are) seen in common, with the speciality knowledge and skills syllabi being the main differences.

In short, the quality of the relationship between the teacher and learner is central to the quality of education that the learner gains.

Further the teacher's interpretation of the context of learning is significant. The accuracy of this interpretation needs frequent checking out! Teachers' subsequent decisions and actions in respect of a learner are only intelligible (explicable and defendable) afterwards by reference to their own understanding and interpretation of the particular situation. Awareness of the context associated with the specific educational discussion ensures greater sensitivity to the nuances of meaning and the complexity of interpretation supervisors (often unwittingly) engage in as they work with learners.

Thus, these new ways of seeing the learner, the context and the more flexible approach to the curriculum can lead to new roles for the teacher and learner.

New roles for the teacher and learner

Please note that much of this entire section has been taken more or less directly from Fish (2012a) Chapter Six, see also Fish (2015) and Fish et al., (2015a and 2015b).

In the moral mode of educational practice, the teacher works with (not on) the learner, and in doing so meets that learner as a whole person. Here, learners are not buckets to be filled nor are they banks into which to deposit the teacher's wisdom, or even actors to be offered critique or feedback on what they did. Instead learners are parties to a dialogue, and with their teacher's help, they need to make their own meaning out of new knowledge gained or an event experienced and recorded. Indeed, they are far more persuaded by exploring for themselves and using under guidance the knowledge on offer, than simply being told. And they benefit better from the visible evidence offered by an observer of the event they have been engaged in, so that through reflection on this, they can come to their own recognition of what occurred. Within this approach they will also find both their achievements and their shortcomings easier to accept than they would if told about them in a 'take it or leave it' fashion that can seem confrontational even when it is not intended to be so.

This is a serious change of role for both teacher and learner. It springs from an understanding that a teacher in the moral mode of practice cultivates learners, engages them in building for themselves new understanding and develops their sensitivities to people and events, rather than acting as a transmitter of information which a poor or difficult learner may then treat as mere adverse opinion. This liberates them, so that they can both become teachers and learners.

The moral mode of practice: a new role for learners and teachers in PGME

The purely technical mode of practice, is what has characterised teaching in PGME over many years and particularly since the beginning of the twenty-first century. Here, the learning doctor is quite simply the object of the teacher's (supervisor's) work! Here, learners are people whose behaviour is to be shaped according to the protocols they are to be trained in, or whose knowledge can be added to through what Freire (1970) has called 'the banking concept' of education. Thus, in the technical mode of educational practice, learners feature less in the teacher's thinking and in their preparation than does the protocol to be taught or the knowledge to be handed on. It is not that the teacher in this mode does not care at all for the learner. Indeed, the teacher may well believe that it is in the learner's best interests to be treated in this way and provided thus with these new skills or knowledge. It is simply that often more thought is given during the teacher's preparation — to what the teacher will do — rather than what the learner will do and who they are as a person, (what they know, how they think, and what their personal qualities and character are). Thus, for the teacher in the technical mode, the 'educational' intentions are focused on what that teacher will do to the learner.

In this technical mode, learners almost become a blank sheet on which the technically-oriented teacher expects to write. Worryingly, many consultants and senior clinicians who teach their learners knowledge and skills in the clinical setting, still broadly (if unconsciously) adopt this approach. This process, sometimes referred to as 'the transmission of knowledge', brings with it, insidiously, an attitude to learners that places them in a passive and unthinking role, and takes little account of them as people.

Freire shows clearly in his work (1970 and 1998/2001) that a 'traditional transmission pedagogy' (the banking approach of imparting the teacher's knowledge into the learner's storage system) can involve learners 'banking' knowledge that is alien to (incompatible with) their normal ways of thinking and understanding, because they have not made meaning out of it for themselves. However, this is not to suggest that the teacher should never be involved in 'transmission'. Further, as Carr, D., (2003) shows, the teacher can also be a 'transmitter of moral values' (by modelling and inviting consideration of that model), but here the intention is not to deposit knowledge but to offer examples from the teacher's own practice for consideration and critique.

By contrast, in the moral mode of practice, learners have a new role. Each one is quite simply the centre of their teacher's focus and the main subject of the teacher's study. Indeed, no educationally worthwhile intentions can be formulated without looking carefully at every aspect of what the learner brings as a person to the educational interaction. Learners then become for the teacher an interest in themselves, a person with whom the teacher can interact collaboratively by means of a learning conversation, such that (normally) both become teachers and learners, and both benefit from greater enjoyment of the process (although learners in difficulty may sometimes need some additional approaches).

Understanding the role of talking and writing for learning

The quality of language used by both teacher and learner shapes the quality of the education provided. How the supervisor uses language in education will determine what the supervisee actually gets from their time with their teacher. By language here we mean both talking and writing (and therefore of course, listening and reading).

The importance of talk in learning

Where the teacher simply and only presents ideas and the learner just listens, (*presentational talk*), little real learning is likely to occur, and even where the learner asks the odd question, this does not of itself constitute evidence of serious learning. Indeed, wherever the teacher does most of the talking, where all the learner is contributing is "Um" or "Yes", all that can be ascertained is that the teacher has the knowledge but no one can know what the learner has learnt. We have many recordings of supervisor/supervisee learning conversations which demonstrate this. As we shall see shortly, this is also true when the teacher gives 'feedback' alone, as there is no real evidence of learning because it is also a one-way process.

Education is not about 'putting in' but about 'drawing out' and helping the learner to build understanding. This requires full interaction between both parties. Too often the teacher starts a session by telling, without having a detailed idea of where the learner needs to begin. Only the learner can say and show where the teaching needs to begin and only the learner can show how they have constructed meaning from what they do, hear, read, think. This is known as meaning-making (Alexander, 2004; Barnes, 1995; Mercer, 2000, 1995/2008; Wells, 2009).

Meaning-making

The meaning-making process involves the active transformation by the learner of the information provided by the teacher and other participants in the educational activity. Here, the learner's resulting knowledge (or understanding) is never a copy of what was initially offered, but rather a personal reconstruction. As a result, it may go beyond the initial 'model' offered and learners may add new meanings and solutions to problems and even formulate new problems. These new meanings need to be shared with the teacher, and the teacher needs to listen carefully and respond to them seriously, because however much learners seem to be speaking the same language as the teacher, this does not automatically mean a shared understanding. The process of sharing talk is variously referred to as 'oral interaction', 'dialogue' or a 'professional conversation'. The latter term is the most commonly used.

Professional conversation

By 'professional conversation' then, is meant a discussion between colleagues, members of the same profession, both of whom acknowledge that they are always both a teacher and a learner. This is not a one-way process, in which the senior teacher gives the learner feedback or a critical commentary, neither is it an interrogation by teacher of learner, as in some debriefing processes. These are activities more suitable to the technical mode of teaching. Rather, the professional conversation seeks to develop a critical appreciation of what happened and what is to be learnt from it. Here the senior doctor picks out salient points of the event and leads the learner to formulate an appreciation of what happened by examining that event from a number of perspectives. Thus, the professional conversation in which the learner works with the teacher in a nurturing environment is a cornerstone of education in the moral mode of practice, and teachers who revert to 'feedback' instead, will quickly see the learner becoming defensive and less open to learning.

Using a professional conversation to formulate an appreciation of a clinical (or even an educational) event, involves collaborative analysis and interpretation in which both parties seek to consider the activity from many points of view, balancing pros and cons, seeking to set it in a context that helps to make sense of it, seeing in it meanings beyond the surface and seeing it as representative of something beyond itself. Further, where both teacher and learner share that exploration together and 'egg each other on', then learning really 'catches fire', and the learner owns their new understanding.

Thus, dialogue rather than monologue, lies at the heart of good teaching. Indeed, Alexander (2004) argues that: 'Dialogue is about enabling the learner to locate him/herself within the unending conversations of culture, community and history. With dialogue comes identity'. But, we would argue that the culture of PGME does not normally encourage this and so a supervisor will need explicitly to invite the learner to use talk with them to explore ideas and develop thinking.

All this would suggest that a judicious and *conscious* mixture of presentational and exploratory talk would be most likely to fulfil the needs of giving the learner some information in combination with getting them to use that information more actively through oral and written exploration.

Writing as central to the learning process

Learners will be familiar with the notion that writing is a means of demonstrating the knowledge they already have. They will have done this over many years in written exams. It is known as *presentational writing*. By contrast, the writing that is central to the learning process is *exploratory writing*. Here the learning occurs during the writing.

During the processes of Transformative Reflection the learner will be asked to engage in more writing than is usual in the educational encounters between teacher and learner, and this will be mainly exploratory. The expectation that learners will engage in this should be flagged up to the learner at the contractual start of their attachment. This will mean that the supervisor will need to understand and to reassure learners from the start, about the following:

- this writing will be all about themselves and their chosen case, and thus will be something that any doctor should be able to write
- being mainly exploratory rather than presentational, it will not be regarded as 'right or wrong' (except where theoretical knowledge or clinical action, were clearly inaccurate or inappropriate)
- the learning will occur during the writing and therefore writing is what draws out main learning insights
- there will be different kinds of writing for different purposes and of different lengths during the Transformative Reflective Process
- the writing will be guided and responded to appreciatively and appropriately by the educator, all along the way
- the end result of the final pieces of writing will be useful for a whole range of purposes.

Reassurance can also be offered about all this and motivation can be stirred if the supervisor shares something of their own Transformative Reflective Writing.

Responding to the written work will not be outside supervisors' current experience as clinical practitioners. The content of the writing will be not only about the clinical facts of the case but more wholistically about what the learner understands about being a doctor, how they conduct themselves in the clinical setting and the clinical decisions and judgements they have made. Chapter Six helps with the writing process itself. A teacher and a learner engaging collaboratively in this form of reflective activity will over even one or two cases become much more insightful of each other's thinking and ways of conducting themselves in real practice.

The importance of using assessment to nurture the learner

Please note that this entire section has been largely taken from Fish, 2012a, Chapter Eight, Eleven and Twelve. See also Fish, 2005.

In the practice setting, clinical supervisors who are also teachers are currently required to engage in formal assessment, using 'tools' to 'measure quality' (although of course quality cannot really be measured by numbers)! The focus here is on what is visible and quantifiable. Such formal assessments, being designed to be operated alongside clinical work, mainly assess learners through observation and talk *in situ*, rather than through writing that reflects upon what has happened in practice and their understanding of it. These 'tools' ignore the fact that it is writing that reveals the detail and nuance of the learner's clinical thinking, decision making and professional judgements – which are at the heart of wise medical practice. While it is true that some reflective writing is required to be uploaded onto the learner's portfolio, it is rarely understood and responded to in educational terms.

Formal assessment used in this administrative way currently ignores the facts that:

- assessment is a part of the education process not an outcome of it, and is properly aimed at promoting and engaging the learner in learning to be a doctor
- the great potential of learners' own writing during an attachment is to provide evidence of their achievements in that attachment, of the person they bring to the service of patients and of their increasing insights and understanding, thus demonstrating the improvement in their service to patients
- self-assessment in learning is powerfully motivating and in the longer term will be increasingly required of them, and can arise naturally for a learner from looking back over their earlier writing and identifying for themselves their own growth of understanding.

This means that assessment is in fact more complex than trainers who work in the technical mode of practice recognise.

By contrast to all this, for educators working in the moral mode of practice, assessment is a means of promoting learning, and is inextricably linked with teaching and learning and with learning about the learner. It does not deliver absolute judgements on a learner's achievements and potential (any more than can any other assessment process). But it does offer a more honest and reliable, if less than totally specific, appreciation of the *quality* of the learner's achievements, based on evidence that is transparent and can be reviewed and considered both by those originally involved, and by others who work with the learner later along their educational pathway. This is because such evidence is in words not figures (which are almost meaningless for later readers) and because the words are the learner's own writing, giving direct evidence of their own self-assessment.

Those who see themselves as involved in education rather than training, recognise these subtleties and complexities. They also recognise that the nature of assessment is shaped by how we construe learning and teaching, so that those who see it as a moral enterprise will wish to use it as part of education. They will appreciate that the value of assessment lies in its educational purposes and that these should shape its processes and products rather than being a 'bolt on' outcome.

Further, educators understand that there is no one means of assessment that will provide the whole picture of a person; of all that they can achieve; of all that they bring to their practice and of all that they have to offer as a professional. That is, there is no one single overall idea which will resolve all the conflicts within the decision making about what to assess, how to assess it and what kind of evidence to seek. In fact, we need a range of assessments (using different forms and from different perspectives) if we are to capture wide enough evidence to be able to talk realistically about the achievements of a human being. This means we need assessment to be derived from: accounts of practice recorded in numbers as appropriate to quantifying some elements of practice; and some accounts captured in words, which are appropriate to demonstrating the quality of character and thinking of the writer. Data using figures for assessment purpose can only evidence *quantity* where words demonstrate quality.

Yet assessment outcomes are so very powerful, that we treat the evidence from just one assessment event as quite unproblematic and as absolute, and definitive, such that people become unjustly labelled and then believe such labels! Worse, incomplete assessment of this kind provides information upon which many decisions are based, and has far-reaching effects — for individuals, for institutions, for the profession, and even for patients and the public.

If we do engage in assessment as a means of supporting teaching and learning and providing helpful information to teachers and learners along the way, then we can with some confidence also use the same results for gate-keeping, (the process of deciding whether to allow a learner to go through to the next level of career and of learning). That way, we can be fairly sure that we have robust, extensive and detailed evidence to justify the label of professional success or failure, and which is demonstrably fair and persuasive.

In the moral mode of practice therefore, assessment is not just about looking at the visible surface of practice, but should plumb the depths of the professional values, thinking, character, decision making and professional judgements of the learner. It should also take account of the whole person that they bring to their practice of medicine, as is shown in their interactions with patients and colleagues. In this way we will be assessing what we have been teaching and the learner has been developing within the moral mode of practice. Thus, assessment is about:

- looking at the learner's achievements and progress wholistically
- providing information that helps to shape further teaching and learning
- demonstrating the learner's ability to learn
- gaining evidence of the professional judgement of the teacher/assessor
- developing the learner's ability to self-assess
- seeing how the learner has used the opportunities available for learning
- placing on record the learner's patterns of achievement, not using a one-off process to make decisions about a learner's future.

Informal assessment, which goes beyond the official requirements for outcome measures, and is created by the teacher for educational reasons, will promote learning. This can be achieved by making active opportunities within their day-to-day teaching for individual learners to undertake tasks designed by their individual teacher in order to reveal their immediate learning needs, as highlighted by the particular context in which they work. This kind of learning activity is already common practice in PGME, but is clearly not always understood by either party as a *key educational strategy* and sometimes it is misread by learners as designed to catch them out! Such informal assessment used educationally, is a natural part of good teaching and can provide information about learners' current understanding and help the teacher to reconsider their next plans or to reshape their next educational interactions with the learner.

This kind of informal assessment activity is 'off the formal record'. This means that the results are not formally recorded, though teachers may write about them for their learners' eyes only and they may also (along with many other kinds of evidence) use the results indirectly, to inform their judgement when writing the formal report on the learner's achievements during the course of the attachment.

The inescapable significance of the assessor's judgement

It is vitally important to remember that all assessments rely somewhere along the line on the professional judgement of the teacher/assessor. There is no process that can totally rid assessment of subjectivity and even some form of bias. Education is not a science. Learning is neither a scientific nor an incremental process. An individual's learning does not conform to a pre-charted pathway, but happens in fits and starts as they meet personal learning plateaux and unexpected racetracks. Thus, the results of assessment are at best temporary and educational judgement is an inescapable element of the assessment process, even where scripts are machine-marked (because judgement informs how the technology has been set up).

Further, since all learners are different, the stage they have reached at the key assessment points will not be entirely predictable, nor can it accurately predict later success or failure. Thus, no assessment can ever be totally objective and none can be totally accurate. Because of this, 'good assessment practice has to recognise the tentative nature of judgements made about achievements', (Murphy, 2002: 179). This is why Broadfoot speaks of the 'myth of measurement' (Broadfoot, 2002).

Endnote

Equipped with the above understandings, it is now appropriate to turn in the following chapter to the planning and teaching of Transformative Reflection.

Without the underpinning recognition of some important basic principles of teaching, learning and assessment, as provided in this chapter, what follows would merely by 'tips for teachers' – that is, it would be a dangerous list of how to do something very subtle, but without the subtlety and without the basis for thinking for yourself – particularly of how to maintain worthwhile education when things do not go according to plan and there are no further instructions. A simple analogy might be doing a hernia repair as if it could always be following a simple and objective set of instructions and without any underpinning anatomical and other medical knowledge! Constructing do-it-yourself furniture would be another example. Remember: nothing is ever as simple as it seems from the outside!

Chapter Ten

Practical help for teaching the Transformative Reflective Process: thinking like a teacher

Introduction
Why learn to engage in Transformative Reflection?
Planning an educationally worthwhile programme
A short introductory programme for those newly learning TRP
Planning a face-to-face learning event as part of the introductory programme
Planning for a learner experienced in the TRP
Some useful teaching strategies: Using talking and writing
Finally, some evaluative questions for teacher to ask self
Endnote

Introduction

This chapter provides practical help for clinical teachers and supervisors who seek to teach the processes of Transformative Reflection. To get the best out of the chapter, we advise that you should first have completed your own exploration of the reflective process, helped by Part Two, and have also read Chapter Nine. There is nothing like the confidence of having experience of and understanding the process yourself from the inside, as well as taking account of sound educational strategies, to stimulate the interest and attention of learners. Chapter Ten is then an important guide to help you to teach this, in the most educational way possible, bearing in mind the constraints of rotas, emergencies and other service demands.

We attend firstly, to what you need to take account of in enabling learners new to Transformative Reflection to learn its processes and give some detailed advice about planning and teaching. Following this, we offer how you might enable those familiar with the basic TR process to go on and use it for a range of purposes. The last section of the chapter describes a range of strategies for ensuring that the education you offer and the time you use with learners are fully worthwhile.

> You are reminded to warn learners that learning the processes of this kind of reflection, like learning any other procedure that is completely new, initially takes some time, but that once it is familiar it will become a tacit habit of practice and the writing process will come more easily and more smoothly.

To begin then, we offer a reminder of why Transformative Reflection is so important, and thus to highlight the key motivations for learning the process.

Why learn to engage in Transformative Reflection?

The Reflective Practice Toolkit, demonstrates that there are many 'templates' for reflection and that the processes they offer as 'tools' can be used to reflect on anything clinical that occurs in professional practice (AMRC and COPMed, 2018). They do not, however, offer anything designed especially for doctors by doctors and none of the well-known templates they advocate offers any means for looking in depth at the heart of medical practice. That is, they do not attend in detail how to recognise, analyse, critique and appreciate either the ontological factors (their own 'being' and the person they have brought to treat the patient), or the epistemological factors (their decision making and the professional judgements that doctors draw on in every patient case). Indeed, these factors are rarely recognised in detail or articulated and shared in depth with others. Further, the reflective templates offer the reason for engaging in reflection as learning from one piece of practice in order to improve their next piece of practice. But learning is not that simple. Whilst having laudable aims therefore, these templates we believe are not going to transform the mind-set of doctors and so develop their practice for the better.

What is offered in this book deals with the complex and invisible in clinical practice. It has been designed and refined precisely in order to enable doctors to explore *their thinking and their being* in practice. This enables them to find ways of articulating much of what goes on in their heads and hearts, in order to learn from it, to develop it and to share it with a range of appropriate people for a range of educational purposes.

We would argue that for doctors of any grade and experience TRP is useful in that it fosters the ability to make the tacit explicit within a patient case. We have experienced that it:

- improves doctors' *detailed* understanding of their current practice and of themselves in that practice
- enables doctors' thinking and being to be unearthed, critiqued and developed
- provides doctors with a means of being far more articulate about their expertise
- means that doctors can share this expertise far more broadly
- places persuasive evidence on record of the regular exploration and refinement by doctors of their practice
- can be a means of contributing to legal cases, crucial detailed information of a doctor's judgements and of the custom and practice of medicine
- would, shared more widely, enable society, and individuals in it, to understand much better the complexity of doctors' decision making and their human and humane response to clinical events.

In other words, this form of reflection *transforms* doctors' understanding of themselves, their detailed thinking, and the nuances of their practice. It transforms their ability to articulate all this to a wide range of people and to give evidence of who they really are and what they do in real practice. It provides a grasp of how medical practice actually works, for those who need to understand it. It thus has the potential to transform society's understanding of what is involved *inside* medical practice and what it is reasonable to expect from the NHS's human servants.

Planning an educationally worthwhile programme

In our experience, and as curriculum design theory argues (Stenhouse, 1975), a curriculum provides a set of guidelines for teachers, and should therefore be captured within a 'definitive' written document. Such documents are there for teachers to adopt in working with specific learners. They also offer an overview of the key issues to be met by all who follow the guidelines broadly, thus ensuring a degree of commonality across all learning events within a particular learning attachment.

Before setting out to plan or to use a short programme for teaching TRP, it is worth considering the classic components of a written curriculum. It usually falls into three main cohering sections: *an introduction* (where the grounds of all decisions about the programme are set out and a foundation is laid for the design); *a main section* offering the main details of the enactment of the curriculum; and a final section on the management of it. The headings then are as follows. Those in blue are crucial to the short programme that is offered below.

The key headings useful for any curriculum (see also Fish and Coles, 2005)

These headings hold good in planning for an event (one teaching session), a short programme of teaching sessions, or a whole course (which might last an entire attachment), but of course if the event is within and a part of a larger curriculum, then not all the general overall details would need to be repeated within, say, each short programme. This is significant here because a short programme about reflection would need to be embedded within the national curriculum guidelines for a given specialty and stage. The details are as follows.

Introductory matters

- Contextual analysis (what current events and changes have led to the need for this new short embedded programme?)
- Evidence of who was involved in the deliberations about devising the programme (as a committee, a group, or an individual?)
- Clear and agreed definitions of key terms used within the document
- Agreed principles, processes and values which informed the deliberations
- Rationale for the curriculum key choices made, on what basis and for what reason
- Criteria for recruitment to the programme (qualifications and experience required at entry)

- Processes for recruitment to the programme (application form; attendance at interview; paperwork to take to interview etc)

The main details of the curriculum

- General overall educational aims
- Specific intentions / objectives / agenda for learners
- Chosen ways of seeing teaching and learning
- Content / syllabus and other matters to be acquired by the learner
- The balance of depth and breadth of what will educate the learner
- The structure of the content and how the learner meets it: (simple linear structure as indicated here; integrated structure which relates theory and practice in a number of possible ways; a spiral approach, in which the learner systematically revisits earlier learning but at a higher level)
- Statement of resources required by both teacher and learner
- Assessment and its role
- Regulations for progression and provision for failure
- Evaluation, which explores rationale, principles and processes of teaching and learning

Processes for the management of the curriculum

- Administrative and educational structures
- Recruitment and selection regulations and criteria
- Regulations for progression
- Quality assurance procedures

Appendix

Glossary of educational terms and their definitions as used within the document

A short introductory programme for those newly learning TRP

Readers should note before reading this part of the chapter, that:

a. The teacher in this chapter means the senior physician or surgeon (the clinical supervisor), and the learner means their more junior colleague (the supervisee).

b. We have demonstrated in what follows, that the structure of this short programme can fit across a sixteen-week period, leaving enough room for the required elements of the Specialty Curriculum to be attended to by both teacher and learner. This framework could, of course be adjusted to fit your own context.

c. If well prepared for, a face-to-face learning event should be no longer than forty minutes. There are only five such face-to-face learning events in this programme. The learner will work independently for the other learning events.

d. A comfortable pace for this programme is to allow one week for each learning event in the first half of the programme and two weeks in the second half of the programme.

e. TRP will become an important resource for exploring the 'being, knowing, thinking, doing, and becoming' endemic to any practice.

It should also be carefully noted by teachers and learners that the TRP is not a 'thing in itself', but rather a key process and set of fundamental resources for engaging in Case-based Discussion, which is a central means of teaching and learning throughout postgraduate medical education in the UK. (A broad overview of engaging in Case-based Discussion is available on www.Ed4MedPrac.co.uk Resource Paper 4.)

We offer below therefore two key stages that may be used to design this short programme for teaching the TRP to those physicians and surgeons who are new to it or who need to revise it again from the start. They demonstrate how the key headings, marked in blue above, can be used for such a design. Indeed, they would, at the level of principle, work for designing any short teaching programme embedded within the wider formal requirements of each learner's specialty postgraduate curriculum. These provide an essential foundation for a properly disciplined and educationally worthwhile attachment.

The headings are: *Preparation for Teaching and Learning, and Main Learning Events.*

1. Preparation for Teaching and Learning

The following two sections a) and b) need to have been completed before the programme can begin.

a) Separate preparation by teacher and learner one week before the programme begins

Teacher to send learner, prior to the commencement of the programme:

- An introductory note to the programme and a brief personal profile (one side of A4) and a request to receive learner's personal profile (if this has not already happened) before meeting together to record the Learning Agreement.
- A copy of the entire programme with a request to be ready to adjust/discuss and set it into the Learning Agreement.
- A reminder to bring a diary / rota for the attachment in order to be able to agree key dates in the TRP programme.

Learner to prepare before first meeting with teacher, as follows:

- READ all papers sent by teacher

- Prepare and send to your teacher before your first meeting, your personal profile on one side of A4 (unless already previously done)

- Become properly informed about the TRP programme, ready to discuss/adjust its details and set it into your Learning Agreement.

b) Setting up the programme together: agreeing the Learning Agreement

1. Discuss TRP, its purposes and values, rationale and educational philosophy.

2. Talk through Table 3.10.1 below and discuss, clarify and agree the programme, activities involved (like engaging in reflective writing), and the importance of roles and responsibilities and of agreeing dates and submitting written work.

3. Clarify the following key matters at the start of the programme:

   a) Both teacher and learner have a responsibility to fulfil their roles in time, in order for this to become worthwhile education.

   b) The basis of this programme sets a different relationship between teacher and learner where the teacher mostly becomes guide and facilitator, rather than instructor and leader, and the learner takes responsibility for writing about their view of the patient case and understanding and critiquing their role in it. The teacher of course remains the arbiter of medical accuracy and good practice.

   c) The programme is a sound example of the discipline necessary for learning as a postgraduate doctor at level seven.

4. Set the following work to be completed before Learning Event 1 (agree this date):

   a) Read: Chapters One (for a contextual analysis of current medical practice), and Chapter Nine, (which provides a guide to teaching and learning in the moral mode of practice), and be ready to discuss them.

   b) Choose a clinical case you and your teacher have agreed to share, think it through and write the key bullet points that summarise it on one side of A4. See Chapter Five for guidance.

The main Learning Events are shown in Table 3.10.1. This table should be read across the book crease. It contains learning events one to nine. The two events that finalise the programme are aimed at ensuring that the learner has summarised their learning experience in this programme and that this has been refined and agreed with the teacher before anything is recorded in their portfolio.

As many surgeons know, it is valuable to 'rehearse in your head' before an operation, the principles of procedure for the process, even though any given case might not proceed in the ways expected! The same is true of an educational programme that is worthwhile. Both teacher and learner benefit from having a sense ahead of:

- the aims, intentions
- the content and logic of the programme
- the roles to be played by each party
- the resources to be used
- the assessment processes.

Readers are therefore encouraged to walk carefully through the path charted by the Table 3.10.1 which demonstrates that although there are nine learning events, only the purple columns require the supervisor's presence, face-to-face with the learner for formal teaching purposes. The text indicates what could perhaps happen in the face-to-face learning event.

An equally important element of the programme is that the learner works independently on four occasions (shown by the white columns that alternate between the purple ones). This independent learning is guided by the wording in the white columns.

The whole programme will include agreed hand-in dates, and an agreed understanding that completing the independent learning work and sending written work in before any face-to-face event, are both essential to enable the teacher to expand what the learner has already understood whilst alone.

Planning a face-to-face learning event as part of the introductory programmme

This section provides outline headings for planning an individual learning event ready to be shared by teacher and learner together. It is merely a more detailed plan than is found within the table above. A plan for a face-to-face learning event enables a teacher to think more clearly and in more detail about how to orchestrate the session. It also encourages teachers to be clear about what learning should be achieved in the session. The teacher should consider how to: plan the session in short phases that link logically together; help the learner to see where the session is going; and ideally engage the learner in different activities during those phases that will help them remember the key learning points. Do not waste time in a session on matters that the learner can explore independently or read in a textbook.

Table 3.10.1 A Programme of Learning Events for teaching TRP to new learners
(NB: The first column of all (in grey) acts for both pages. Purple indicates teacher and learner working together, white shows learner working independently.

Learning events 1 week apart

The Learning Pathway Curriculum Requirements	Learning Event 1	Learning Event 2	Learning Event 3	Learning Event 4
Learning Intentions for each Event Teacher (T) Learner (L)	Dialogic session to check understanding: - of readings - appropriateness of case selected - review accuracy of bullet point of the case - of how to enrich the narrative Chapter Five	L to work on enriching the bullet points helped by prompts in Chapter Six	Dialogic discussion on L's experience of doing the process and the new insights they have had about the case, themselves and what they need to learn further	L to work independently to enrich narrative with **Invisibles Four, Five & Six** See Chapter Six
Content	L to bring bullets of chosen case and notes from reading and to present these T to draw out understanding of the whole enterprise L to leave with agreed case and bullets and ready to work on enriching the bullets using **Invisibles 1, 2 & 3** Chapter Six Agree date for T to receive writing	L works alone using the prompts Send to T on agreed date T reads L's work and prepares response and all other needs for next session	L offers how it went and asks any questions necessary T responds to L's offerings and then to the writing, Ensures its clinical accuracy, drawing out L's new insights and adding to them Together they set up L's work on **Invisibles 4, 5 & 6** Agree date for T to receive writing	L works alone on **Invisibles 4 - 6** & writes responses & then reviews all narrative Sends to T on agreed date T reads L's work and prepares response for next session, and also to discuss narrative as whole & introduce interrogating the narrative Chapter Seven
Resources	Bullet points Chapter Five	L to decide on digital or hand written text. (see Chapter Five) L needs Chapter Six & Bullet points	Both need a copy of the narrative so far with the T's comments Chapter Six	Chapter Six L needs copies own writing & Chapter Seven
Roles of Teacher & learner at each event	L to start / T to respond in discussion T respond to L's writing Together discuss enriching the bullet points and prepare for next Invisibles	L works alone and sends work in T reads work ahead of meeting and responds	L to start orally & T to respond T respond to L's writing Together prepare for next Invisibles	L works alone and sends in whole enriched narrative T reads work ahead of meeting and prepares for it
Agreements/ Assessment/ Records/Prep for the next Learning Event T responsible for keeping written contemporaneous notes on L's development	Informal: T to share notes on progress Self-assessment L L to enrich the bullet points using chapter Six	Self-assessment by L on what new insights they had during the writing	Informal: T to share notes on progress L to make notes on what they have gained during the process	Written self-assessment by L on what new insights they had during the writing

Learning events 2 weeks apart

Learning Event 5	Learning Event 6	Learning Event 7	Learning Event 8	Learning Event 9
Review all, & prepare for Interrogation of narrative using **Invisibles 7 & 8** Chapter Seven	Interrogate the enriched Narrative using the three processes described in Chapter Seven	Dialogically discuss means of interrogating the narrative and **L's** written responses to them Link with other cases in practice Agree date for **T** to receive writing	Learner works on summative statement See Chapter Eight	Discuss summative statement Refine summative statement Agree next professional development (to go to next attachment) Agree date for **T** to receive writing
L offers how it went and asks any questions necessary **T** responds to **L's** offerings and then to the writing, drawing out **L's** new insights and adding to them Together they set up **L's** work on interrogating the narrative Agree date for **T** to receive writing	**L** works independently and sends in responses on agreed date **T** reads work ahead of meeting and prepares for it	What has been learnt from interrogating the case and preparing for the summative statement	**L** works alone using all that has been learnt so far and may consider sending a new case to **T** on an agreed date This will depend on progress to date and other commitments	**L's** statement to be explored and agreed List of further professional development needed
Both need a copy of writing Chapters Six and Seven	Chapter Seven and **L's** writings	Chapter Eight	Chapter Eight Various drafts of the narrative	All up to date papers
L to start orally & **T** to respond **T** respond to **L's** writing Together prepare for the interrogation Informal: **T** to share notes on progress **L** to make notes on what they have gained during the process	**L** needs copies own writing & the next Invisibles and the prompts Written self-assessment by **L** on what new insights they had during the writing	**L** to start / **T** to respond in discussion **T** respond to **L's** writing Create list of comments on the type and quality of the clinical thinking by the **L** in this case Informal: **T** to share notes on progress **L** to make notes on what they have gained during the process	**L** needs to collate all work to date and complete a draft of the summary of new understandings and learning during this programme and to use this to plan further teaching and learning sessions Written self-assessment by **L** on what new insights they had during the writing and how this has influenced their everyday clinical practice	**L** introduces summary statement and joint discussion then follows. Learner to be clear about **T's** view of progress Semi-formal: **T** to summarise their new and deepening insights about **L's** developing clinical thinking and understanding of their roles and capability as a doctor

What follows is an outline plan for any single learning event within the above programme where learner and teacher work together. You should insert your own detail in place of any specialty specific references.

Table 3.10.2 Planning a Learning Event to be attended by both the teacher and the learner

Face-to-face Event 'X'	Date 'Y' Duration 40 minutes
Overall aims of the programme	To enable the learner to become confident in the process of TRP as a professional discipline for postgraduate doctors
Intentions of the specific event	Say here what you intend that the learner will experience / achieve / understand today as a result of detailed scrutiny of the work they sent ahead
Resources needed	List the resources you need to take with you to the learning event. List what the learner needs to bring (alert them beforehand)
Structure of Learning Event	4 phases as below

Phase One (ten minutes)
1. Share with learner and negotiate your key specific learning intentions, *for this learner*, today.
2. Show that you value the work the learner has sent you and will use it as the basis of the learning event (but only as appropriate)! If no work was sent in, send learner away and record this formally and the reason for it and arrange a new date.
3. Ask learner to share their new understanding of where they are and what they have done and what questions they now have about the work they sent in.
4. Pick up points necessary as learner's knowledge and understanding require.
5. Probe for further meaning-making by the learner.

Phase Two (ten minutes)
6. Link this work today to whole sequence of the curriculum for learning TRP.
7. Explore the work produced by learner which you have already scrutinised and support and enhance / extend the thinking it contains, through oral

discussion in which learner takes the larger part.
8. Learner to link main topic of discussion (these ideas / questions / writing) with other clinical events you have shared in practice.
9. Probe further for new insights about professional and clinical matters as guided by the learner's specific national curriculum — including the humanistic/professional aspects as well as the clinical facts and principles.

Phase Three (ten minutes)
10. Get the learner to summarise the key learning points and if necessary probe and uncover anything missed.
11. Ask the learner what key clinical points they will now take away from this event.
12. Ask the learner what they have learnt about themselves in this event.

Phase Four (ten minutes)
13. Draw to a conclusion / talk about next session / check anything else needed.
14. Discuss how learner's achievements are to be turned into evidence of progress and new understanding.
15. Send Learner away with clear work to do and a clear date to do it by: To follow up this event and prepare for next learning event.
16. Evaluation by the learner at the end of the event:
    What new understanding they have I come to?
    Were the learning intentions appropriate for me?
    How did the learning intentions work out for me?

Assessment process	Indicate what you think will be the best way of assessing the learner's achievements (be prepared to adapt this if necessary). For example: should the learner have gained other insights and new understandings in addition to those intended, these should be duly acknowledged and recorded as part of the assessment records.
Reminders to Teacher	Think about the following as you plan.

- How to word the questions you use for the key points you need to make, so that they are not intimidating but supportive.

- How you will respond if Learner gets it wrong and how far you will praise them if it's correct.

> - How will you probe for further understanding and where in the event is that likely to come?
>
> - How much information / knowledge / understanding you will expect from this learner. Have high but appropriate expectations and articulate them. Hope to be surprised!

Such planning, once done can be a useful basis for all future learning events, though it may need to be adapted to each learner, on each occasion.

Planning for a learner experienced in the TRP

Before engaging in using TRP for a variety of educational purposes, a learner experienced in the processes should nonetheless be asked to remind themselves of the key procedures for TRP, by reading Part Two of this book.

When teaching doctors, who are more experienced in using TRP, the processes are almost entirely dialogic and again the quality of the learning here is dependent on the quality of the questions being asked of the writer about the nuances and underlying tones of their oral and written work. The questions found in Chapters Seven and Eight above may be a starting point for the teacher. Thus the plan for teaching in this way needs to ensure that the structure and timing of the professional conversation that should occur, uses the same structure as shown in Table 3.10.2 above.

It will soon become clear that the focus of the writing emanating from more experienced doctors explores the more humanistic elements of being a doctor, emphasising their *being*, rather than simply exploring the epistemological facts of a case. The importance of this process therefore is not just to teach facts but for teacher and learner to understand each other's thinking better and so to help the less experienced doctor to grow in understanding and confidence and thus not only be more capable but also a more efficient and useful practitioner.

As an experienced physician or surgeon, you will see things quickly in what a less experienced doctor writes. You do not have to learn anything new to do this. In fact you do it already in your observation of their practice and how they seem to perform as a practitioner. Rarely is this performance explored by the learner in such detail that has been offered here. One or two cases, shared together, will cement the teacher/learner relationship and where the learner does most of the interrogation of their writing they will be offering their own critique of their practice. Again such writing often brings up topics that do not usually feature in a scheduled list of teaching events. We offer one such example from recent practice below.

What follows is one very small section of a piece of Rainbow Writing, done as part of a routine teaching and learning programme designed by Linda to explore thinking and decision making. There was no complaint or criticism of the case. The focus was the event of a night on call. Linda reports: "I read the whole piece offered by the doctor. It was well done and she had attended to the task well. Two things struck me and I have italicised them below."

> *In order to be more efficient, I asked my SHO to start in A&E and I reviewed the first patient on the night shift who was already being transferred to the surgical admission Unit. I also continued monitoring the situation on the emergency list as I wanted to stay up-to-date about the availability of slots. The plastic surgeons had already been in theatre for a good two hours trying to save a flap and there was no end in sight. Rumours of an incarcerated inguinal hernia started emerging.* (Extract from the narrative from a surgeon in training.)

Linda then continues: "When I met with the writer I chose to start our discussions as follows, after our usual introductory greetings".

LdeC	'I am pleased to see that you were making logistical decisions to manage the busy night and that is pretty routine but I wonder if you could tell me what things go through your mind when you delegate to a more junior colleague?'
Doctor	'Mmmm that's an interesting point I have never thought about that in detail…..

Our conversation continued around this subject. The next session we had together, the trainee related that she had gone on thinking about this and the next time she delegated she had taken time to talk to the junior doctor in more detail to ensure that her decision to delegate was sound. This is an example of how the TRP was influencing (very quickly) the young surgeon's thinking in everyday practice.

The learning opportunity I had seen here was to raise awareness of the responsibility of the delegating doctor to ensure that this was indeed a safe decision. Such conversations do not usually happen.

Linda continues: "My second learning opportunity was about professionalism across specialities in theatre! It was to emphasise that irritation at being kept waiting for operating space in theatre, which is not an uncommon phenomenon at night, (and which did seem to be showing through in the writing) only heightens tensions all around and often prevents satisfactory solutions and ways forward to alleviate the problem. Our conversation continued productively again along a pathway that the trainee had not expected but found most helpful and informative".

What this professional conversation between teacher and learner demonstrates is that when the reflective writing is used as a focus of the talking, more can be unpicked about the complex subtleties of practice that are often left to chance or are never explored.

Some useful teaching strategies: Using talking and writing

This section is offered both to those teaching learners new to TRP and those helping learners use it for professional development purposes.

Talking for learning: some useful teaching strategies

> **The two following questions are key to evaluating the language strategies that teachers use:**
>
> Do we provide the right kind of talk to promote *thinking* in our learners? (or do we just ask factual questions to test memory?)
>
> How can we strengthen the power of talk to help learners think and learn, even more effectively than they already do?

A good principle to remember is that *dialogue* between teacher and learner is the best way of extending their thinking while they are with you. There are four forms of dialogue:

- Presentation /exposition
- Discussion
- Question and Answer
- Listening and responding

What we offer here are some strategies for dialogic teaching. You will find you are instinctively using most of these, so the point of this sub-section is more to enable you to become conscious of what you do, so that you can develop it. We also offer you here the language in which to talk and think about teaching.

Dialogic Teaching sees teaching as:

- **collective**: teacher and learner address learning tasks together
- **reciprocal**: teacher and learner listen to each other, share ideas, consider alternatives
- **supportive**: learners articulate their ideas freely, without fear of embarrassment over wrong answers, and also help each other with common understandings
- **cumulative**: teacher and learner build on their own and each other's ideas and chain them into coherent lines of thinking and enquiry
- **purposeful**: teachers plan and facilitate dialogic teaching with particular educational aims and intentions in view.

Dialogic teaching takes the view that knowledge and understanding come from testing evidence, analysing ideas, and exploring values, rather than unquestioningly accepting somebody else's certainties. The following list offers the kinds of strategies that teachers have found important to consider. These are useful touchstones in three situations: when planning teaching; when actually engaged in it; and when evaluating it afterwards.

Some strategies to prompt learners to think

1. Engage in collaborative activities and seek to help the learner to collaborate with you in talking something through.
2. See as much of your teaching as possible as a joint enquiry.
3. See talk as one main means of developing the learner's thinking and reasoning.
4. Use the things the learner 'has to do' to engage him/her in talking about their thinking.
5. Press the learner a little harder, probe the response, wait — and don't answer for them!
6. Ask 'authentic questions' (those for which the teacher has not pre-specified the answer).
7. Ask questions that elicit reasoning and speculation.
8. Question in order to promote discussion; clarify to tackle problems in understanding; summarise what has been learnt before you move on – and get the learner to do this summary; encourage the prediction of what will follow.
9. Give learners time to think aloud – don't jump in and answer for them.
10. Recognise the difference between 'interactive pace' and 'cognitive pace'. Thinking takes longer than talking! Learners rush in to show you that they are awake. Show them that you value their stopping and thinking, rather than just rushing in.
11. Show that you are a good and careful listener. Respond to their agenda, not yours.
12. There is little point in framing a well-conceived question and giving the learner ample 'wait time' to answer it, if we fail to engage with the answer given and hence the understanding or misunderstanding that it reveals.
13. Think about when an informal conversational style of talk is appropriate, and when something more precise and formal is necessary… and use this distinction! (this is about *register* – the tone of voice and choice of vocabulary appropriate to a situation).
14. Order your talking logically and pace your time with learners so as to get the most out of oral interaction with them.

Many of the supervisors Della has encouraged to record their teaching and listen to it, have discovered that although they think they are doing all these things well, in fact they are not. Quite a few have found that they have not responded at all appropriately to what a learner has said and even have agreed with an answer that is incorrect. This mistake is easier to make than you might believe!

Use the following to think about your responses to supervisees and others who learn with you.

- A teacher's response to learners' answers gives informative diagnostic feedback on which the learner can then build. Do not just say 'yes' or 'no'. Do not just repeat the answer.
- Use reformulation to indicate clearly the quality of the answer (where it is in some way lacking).
- Use praise discriminatingly.
- Keep lines of enquiry open rather than closing them down.
- Set an atmosphere in which learners can articulate their ideas without fear of embarrassment.

Writing for Learning (see also pages 94-97)

This section is merely to remind teacher/supervisors and tell learner/supervisees that we have already made the point that writing can be presentational (in which what has already been learnt by the learner is presented as evidence of their current knowledge); or exploratory (in which the learning is in the writing and the whole process reveals many new perspectives to consider). In Transformative Reflection, much of the writing is exploratory such that the process of setting down a narrative and then interrogating it for further tacit meanings, beliefs and understanding, *is the main activity for the learner.*

This means that the teacher needs to respond promptly, thoughtfully and sensitively to what the learner has produced and to help them build on it. The content of such a response will be obvious, being about either the expected level of the learner's understanding and insight of clinical practice and/or a response to the learner as a person. The tone and nuance of what the teacher writes or says in response however, may need to be carefully modulated to the needs and personality of that particular learner. Once alerted to this, the teacher should be able to draw on common sense in deciding how to respond in a way that will lead to openness and learning rather than defensiveness and a learning block.

The early draft(s)

The following offers some things to think about in seeking to help learners to refine or re-draft their first draft.

1. The learner needs to attend to the voice of their text

The relationship between writer, subject and audience is what shapes writing. The voice of the text is the personal sound of how the writer communicates with their reader, which in turn affects how the reader sees the writer and the subject. The following are the key things that give an individual voice to writing:

> The tone of the writing: the way the words come over because of what is emphasised and the attitude to the subject.

The written style: the shape and length of the sentences that are used, and the specific nuance of the vocabulary that is chosen.

The form: the overall way the writing is structured and ordered and the logic in what is said.

2. Reflective writing needs to be vivid and enable the reader to 'be there'

It is about concrete situations and 'is in the moment', offering the reader a real sense of being there.

It seeks to study an event/action more deeply and to unpack the thinking and knowing beneath its surface.

It is narrative in style.

It attends in detail to the context of the action/event being reflected on.

It sometimes uses figurative language (rich descriptions based on, for example, comparisons using similes and metaphors).

3. The story is substantially personal and needs to be both descriptive and revealing of the writer's thoughts at the time and their beliefs and attitudes

This means that the writer should:

write in the first person singular

write about their own practice, not someone else's

show evidence of their learning (deepening understanding)

demonstrate their commitment to professional ideals and use these as a touchstone to critique their own practice (my values are X but I did Y)

take account of the views and perspectives of others involved in the action or event

identify the factors contributing to the situation — which may be historical, political, economic, social, ethical, autobiographical, and psychological

draw attention to what may previously have been taken for granted, rendering the familiar strange

offer experience as enriched by the acquisition of new perspectives.

Thus, the writer should work over their narrative so that they tell it in a voice that is alive, personal, and open, in a style that is engaging, in words that are appropriately vivid and in a tone that is professional, friendly and yet intrigued / interested / surprised.

When the piece of writing has been completed, the writer should read it aloud and make any final small corrections as they go. Joint teacher/learner decisions should be made about whether this piece should be presented in the learner's portfolio and with or without the colours of Rainbow Writing. The learner should make sure it is dated and has a title. A summary should also be submitted by the learner demonstrating what this case specifically says about their growing expertise, professionalism and self-knowledge.

In collecting and presenting several dated pieces of reflective writing, each associated with a particular period of time (an attachment for learners, or a year for appraisees, for example), it becomes possible to identify quite quickly some important patterns. These will include developments in skill, knowledge, understanding and insight, and about the writer's clinical expertise and professionalism, as evidenced (or not), across the pieces. Such a record is also helpful in pinpointing a problem if a doctor is in difficulty, clinically or professionally.

The Assessment of reflective writing

All responses from a supervisor about a supervisee's work are, in one way or another, a form of assessment. We believe that all assessment should contribute to worthwhile education and so should be part of the learning processes. Some responses from the supervisor will aim to provide informal assessment, which in this context is mainly a means of working with the learner to extend or improve a draft of the writing. This draft is not made public in any way. In informal responses to drafts, the aim is not 'to mark' it as a teacher might. Rather, we should seek to construct an appreciation of its qualities as a piece of writing designed to communicate vividly with readers who 'have not been there.'

The formal assessment is made only of the finalised writing. We would argue that this assessment of reflection should attend to the quality of the clinical content, the quality of the learner's self understanding and the quality of the writing. Assuming that all supervisors will easily analyse the quality of the learner's clinical practice, and the early drafts of the writing, we offer here some ways of both exploring and assessing the finalised version for the writer's ability to convey their thinking in writing, and to comment on the quality of that writing. The following questions should help you in this.

Questions to consider during formal assessment

The bolded questions are the key ones, the others are prompts to help you think further.

What are your first impressions about the doctor who has written this case?

> What gives the writing its 'credibility'?
> Does the writing make you want to read to the end?
> How has this been achieved?
> What are the writer's key values and priorities (what does the writer 'stand for')?
> What does the writer say overtly about themselves?
> What can reasonably be deduced about them?

How would you describe the writer's voice and attitude to their subject?

> How do we learn about 'the person the writer is'?
> Is what the writer says confirmed or contradicted by the way that they say it?
> What gives the piece its structure and how does that help the reader understand what is being said?
> How helpful, to the writer and to the reader, in understanding the case, are the original bullet points?
> How are those bullet points now being used in the main piece?
> How are you helped as reader to find your way through the writing?
> What do the colours highlight about the doctor and the case?
> In what order do you meet the information? (Chronological or not?)
> How clearly is the writing set out, and how well does it flow?
> Is it technically accurate, linguistically? Why does this matter?

How does the author meet and take account of the reader?

> Does the writer overtly acknowledge and take account of the reader and their needs?
> What are the key means of doing this?
> By what means does the writer make the case vivid for the reader?
> How do you know that this is the doctor's personal voice?
> What further information / comment would you like to have been offered?
> What do you discern as a fellow professional about the needs of this writer?

Readers should note that we have placed this sub-section on assessment at the end of our comments on reflective writing, because we do not regard any one assessment process as capable of providing an overall label for a learner, and believe that all responses to written work should be 'appreciative' and encouraging rather than over-critical and punitive.

Finally, some evaluative questions for teacher to ask self

Teachers too need to learn to improve their practice by reflecting on it. It is often worth getting the help of evaluations from several perspectives in order to get a more realistic view. For example, learner's evaluations of their learning experience may be less enthusiastic straight after the event than later when they begin to see more of where the work is going, can recognise the care taken in structuring the phases of their learning, and also have had time to see how it relates to their practice. Thus, in addition to asking yourself the following self-evaluation questions, it is important to gain perspectives from your learners.

Some useful self-evaluation questions

1. Did I listen properly to the learner?
2. Did I outline the intentions for today's learning event clearly and did the learner agree to it?
3. Was the order of events / phases logical?
4. What do I need to check on again with the learner?
5. Were my questions short and to the point?
6. Was the face-to-face event properly dialogic?
7. What am I pleased with about my own role today?
8. What most pleased me about the learner today?
9. What do I need to remember in my next planning

Finally, remember that teaching and providing education (like medical practice) are both open capacities and that we all go on learning to refine and improve our work throughout our careers. See Fish et al., (2015c).

Endnote

This book has offered a background to reflection (Part One), a methodology for senior doctors for learning TRP (Part Two) and a process of teaching this (Part Three). The final section will offer a vision for the future of how to take this work further.

Part Four

Reaching for the Future

Introduction to Part Four

We began this book by exploring, in Part One, the context, and the historical and current traditions of Reflective Practice, as used in a wide range of professions. We then moved in Part Two, to demonstrate a new way of engaging with the process of reflection, as designed and developed in detail, especially for medical practitioners. Here, we had in mind the importance of reclaiming our professionalism, practical wisdom (sound decision making and good professional judgement), and the moral agency of professionals as needed in today's professional practice. In Part Three, we looked at the traditions of education as a practice, and set out clearly how to teach TRP within the moral mode of educational practice, so that even skeptical learners can come to see it as worthwhile education.

Throughout these Three Parts, we have attempted to show that TRP is a truly educational process, in that it can sharpen a doctor's acumen (their ability to make good judgements and take quick decisions) and enable them to articulate for themselves and develop further, the deepest elements of what characterises their professional practice. The first six of our proposed long-term aims (see above p. 3) have been concerned with the development of medical practice and the improvement of the education of medical practitioners. The final goal was:

> vii. To have the courage to lead their profession and the public they serve to understand the need to slough off the limited conditioning of the target-driven agenda, of seeing all motivation in negative, power-generated and greed-driven terms and to be open to the potential power of unconditional love.

In order to fulfil this long-term aspiration, we expressed the last two of our intentions in this book as:

> vi. to indicate how, when shared, this can contribute towards the reinstatement of the standing of professionals in the eyes of the public, the main professional bodies and the government

> vii. to open up, in the final section of the book, some further avenues for exploration and research into Transformative Reflection.

Having reviewed them carefully it seems to us that these aspirations and immediate intentions are a reasonable basis from which to complete our argument about providing greater understanding about how doctors think and how they might be better educated, for a wider range of laypersons and professionals other than medical practitioners and also to open out a space for further creative developments that might enrich the exploration of TRP.

In Chapter Eleven, the first of two chapters in Part Four, we therefore make the case at the level of principle, that sharing our thinking and experience across professions where each maintains it own uniqueness is a way of deepening our own professionalism and respecting that of others. We believe that this means sharing (through Rainbow Writing about anonymised cases), the complexity and special nature of medical practice with those both inside and outside medicine, who need to understand it better. We believe, that when shared, this writing and its associated talking will also benefit society's understanding of how doctors think and act, and thus clarify what it is reasonable to expect from The NHS's human servants. We end by making a plea for educational research into reflective practice in medicine and offer principles for all other professions beyond healthcare.

In the final chapter of the book, we open up the possibility of there being more Invisibles. We do so by proposing as a new Invisible the idea of the wisdom of the heart which might be brought finally to check out the whole enriched case for its spiritual qualities. This involves creating a new heuristic, as readers will see.

Throughout all this, our guiding light is the quotation placed at the very start of this book:

Practices are changed by changing the way in which they are understood.
Carr, W., Kemmis, S. (1986: p 91)

Chapter Eleven

A wider perspective on the value and use of The Transformative Reflective Process: understanding each other's thinking

Introduction
Physicians and surgeons understanding themselves: why and how?
Physicians and surgeons sharing their thinking with others: why and how?
The Vital need for Researching Reflective Practice as a means of developing Medical Practice
The implications for other professions beyond healthcare
Endnote

Introduction

In Part One of this book, we made the point that doctors rarely make explicit the thinking that underpins their decision making. We believe that maturing professionals need to be able to articulate more cogently, not only their specialist knowledge and clinical thinking but their own sense of vocation, along with their motivations, identity, professionalism and moral agency. To mature this fully it needs to become a habit of mind. Few understand this innately. It needs to be intentionally taught, learnt and practised. This is important to ensure that fellow professionals, people they work with and in particular patients, understand them better.

The Transformative Reflective Process, described in this book, is a resource that has been designed specifically with physicians and surgeons in mind which when learned intentionally as part of their professional development, will allow them to come to know themselves better, be able to strengthen their professional character and practice and if shared, become understood better, by those they work with and those they teach.

This penultimate chapter then goes on to link our ideas with those icons of wise medical practice from the past. Our extensive experience of the last twenty years in researching, teaching and refining our own understanding of 'why' and 'how' physicians and surgeons should reflect on their practice underpins our efforts to make this possible.

Our better understanding of the role of reflective practice in medicine, gained by teaching hundreds of senior professionals about this matter, has strengthened our resolve about its benefits when used educationally and continues to widen our thinking about the deep influences of the tacit elements of our being as professionals, which we share in more depth in the final chapter of the book.

Physicians and surgeons understanding themselves: why and how?

William Osler, former Regius Professor of Medicine at Oxford, extolled to new medical graduates in 1889 at the University of Pennsylvania medical graduation ceremony, that the most important quality of a physician or surgeon was *Imperturbability* '... *coolness and presence of mind under all circumstances, calmness amid storm, clearness of judgment in moments of grave peril, immobility, impassiveness, or, to use an old and expressive word, phlegm*'. (Osler, 1889) He went on to say that this was the quality most appreciated by the laity and without it the doctor loses the confidence of his patients. He believed that this characteristic was innate and divinely endowed. You either had it or you didn't. As a result the medical curriculum at the time and even to this day, does not contain educational resources or teaching, to support the development of this vital characteristic.

The second essential quality he saw was *Equanimity*, which he categorised as the mental equivalent to *Imperturbability*. He said this was difficult to obtain! He offered no real way of learning for this except the important advice that graduates should reflect on their own foibles and those of their patients. Current curricula and postgraduate medical education still have not grasped the need to make the development of such qualities the core of the development of wisdom in medical practice.

The last forty years has seen such an exponential rise in the great innovations that physicians and surgeons can offer patients. Doctors appear in practice to act with fluency and speed such that to the outsider, their decision making and the arguments for it, which underlie their resulting professional judgements and the actions that emanate from them, are never revealed. Perhaps we have become too good at *Imperturbability*? The current curricula focus on the necessary theoretical knowledge needed and on the complex skills many doctors need to have. Whilst this is very necessary, this learning is almost in exclusion to learning about the tacit influences that drive practice and how to strengthen one's capacity to understand better how these influence that practice. The Transformative Reflective Process has been designed, tested out and refined specifically to support physicians and surgeons in doing this.

In clinical practice, doctors need to strengthen their capacity to act autonomously with the interests of the individual patient in front of them, at all times. The many doctors whom we have worked with, strive vigorously to ensure that their patients get the best care that they can. The assumption that doctors don't see service as part of their professional life is false. It is still there at the heart of their vocation as doctors. What does seem to have happened in the last 40 years, in the name of efficiency, productivity and pace, have obliterated the invisible and unmeasurable elements that underpin wisdom in practice.

Chapter Eleven

Physicians and surgeons sharing their thinking with others: why and how?

In Chapter One we made the point that how doctors think and how they communicate the complexity of their practice to patients and public, is just not well understood. What needs attention is their:

Being a doctor, which is about the whole person they are and how they inevitably bring themselves in entirety to their work;

Thinking as a doctor, which is about their decision making and judgements in respect of patients;

Knowing as a doctor which is about all the generic and specialty knowledge (which is considerably more than textbook) that they bring to their work;

Doing as a doctor is about the skills they engage in and the abilities they harness, in the service of patients;

Becoming a better doctor (de Cossart and Fish, 2005; Fish, 2015a).

These five elements permeate all of the teaching and learning that we support. They help to ensure that the whole doctor is attended to in their continuing education.

The teacher and the learner

Our vision for the future, is that reflection on practice becomes a well-developed habit of continuing professional development for physicians and surgeons because it will deepen the experience and the learning that will emanate from researching and critiquing their everyday practice. As T.S. Eliot said:

"We had the experience but [without reflection on practice we] missed the meaning. And approach to the meaning restores the experience in a different form." T.S. Eliot.

Deep learning comes from honest, rigorous and disciplined investigation of one's own practice. This in turn, nurtures self-knowledge, confidence and the recognition of the un-masterable capacity that is wisdom. In practice it must first be learned under the guidance of a wise teacher. It must be given the respect of time and effort. Written reflection on practice will translate into reflection in practice and will transform the thinking and actions of the doctors who make the effort to do it well.

Hunter said in her book *Doctors' Stories* (1993): 'Medicine is not a science. Instead, it is a rational, science-using, inter-level, interpretive activity, undertaken for the care of a sick person.' Her book makes a strong argument to support this. She quotes Leon Kass, physician, biochemist, ethicist, and Henry Luce, Professor of Philosophy at the

University of Chicago: 'Medicine ... is a fertile ground for understanding "the moral relation between knowledge or expertise and the concerns of life."'

We have come to see the paradox of coping with the binary ends of a spectrum of a desire 'to cure' with being able to offer 'no cure' as the normative position of doctors and their intention to treat their patients. Doctors know in their hearts that there is no absolute certainty of a cure. Many conditions that are part of their responsibility need support and education of their patient, working with them at all times to understand better the means of living with a complex illness. Being able to work in the difficult balancing act between those two extremes is the challenge for all doctors.

Self-understanding and growing self-awareness and a sense of personal authority need to be developed in order to act prudently and wisely in all clinical situations. The ability to examine professional judgements, recognising all the influences that will come to bear on their decision making, is essential to strengthen the doctors' capacity as a trusted practitioner. Coming to recognise and being able to articulate more clearly their clinical decision making and professional judgements, brings more to appreciate in patient care than just knowing the facts. Growing in this wisdom is associated with something that we recognise as inner discernment. We will expand on this in Chapter Twelve.

Indeed, we would argue that if doctors used the Transformative Reflective Process with well-chosen cases and on a regular and intentional basis, their ability to make the tacit explicit within a patient case they have attended to, will become a habit of their practice and in time enable them to think more precisely and wisely during that practice.

This is essential because, as we said in Chapter One, it will:

- improve their *detailed* understanding of their current practice and of themselves in that practice
- enable their thinking and being to be unearthed, critiqued and developed
- provide them with a means of being far more articulate about their expertise
- enable them to share this expertise far more broadly
- place persuasive evidence on record of their regular exploration and refinement of their practice
- be a means of contributing to legal cases, crucial detailed information of a doctor's judgements and of the custom and practice of medicine
- if shared more widely, it should enable society, and individuals in it, to understand much better the complexity of doctors' decision making and their human and humane response to clinical events and patient cases.

We now believe that this final point is as important as the rest as we shall show opposite.

Chapter Eleven

The doctor and the manager

Equipped with a better understanding of their clinical thinking and professional judgements, doctors will have the confidence to share this with managers with whom they work on a daily basis.

Managers, as we in the NHS in the UK know them, are a relatively new professional group. Their development was triggered in 1983, by the Griffiths Report (https://www.bmj.com/content/bmj/287/6402/1391.full.pdf). The nature of their role has become profoundly bureaucratic and their regulatory and controlling role has created an increasingly widening gap between themselves and doctors.

At workshops with NHS managers in the last few years, one of us (LdeC) found that managers in a big hospital felt very separated from their senior medical colleagues. Working with these managers to support their better understanding of their doctors has been both a surprising and rewarding experience. An honest and respectful context established an atmosphere to enable healthcare managers to express how they really saw their consultant colleagues. The results of two brain storming sessions with two different groups of managers is shown in Figure 4.11.1. The themes reflected are also found in the discourse of other managers in healthcare.

The interactive sessions which followed this beginning, were surprising in that how little these intelligent and thoughtful people knew about doctors, about their professional journey to their role as consultants and in particular the time they had been on that journey. They showed respect for their medical colleagues but rarely had an opportunity to get to know them better professionally and in particular to consider the complexity of their roles and the decisions they made. They showed a genuine interest in reading narratives from senior doctors (as described in this book) and were very quickly able to see in these narratives, a completely different side of a senior professional's thinking.

Figure 4.11.1 Results of brainstorming what managers think of doctors

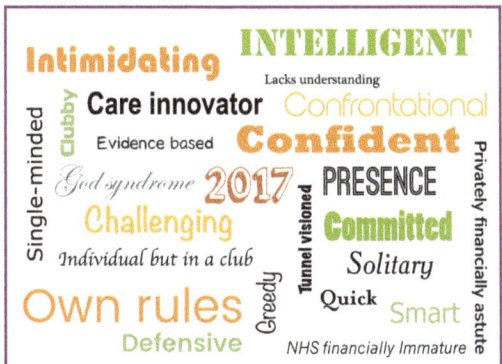
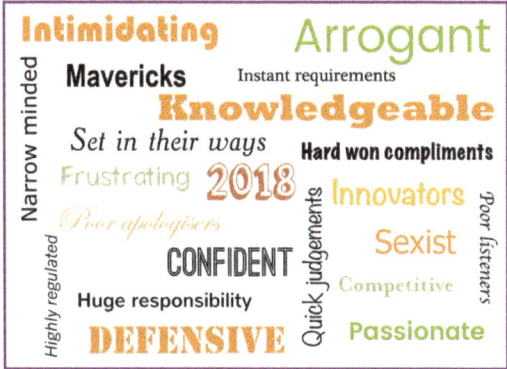

Doctors sharing narratives of their decision making in key cases is a valuable means of better understanding the 'why' and 'how' of doctors visible everyday practice. There is a place for judicious sharing of case narratives between managers and doctors and this activity may well help both to work more productively with each other. The best care of patients deserves such developments.

The doctor, the patient and their relatives

Nowhere is the misunderstanding of the 'why' and the 'how' doctors act, more evident than how they are reported when things go wrong. There is a case for doctors taking responsibility to share with the public the complexities and uncertainties of medical practice. The Transformative Reflective Process we have described, offers a disciplined and rigorous way for doctors to unpack their clinical thinking and the actions (professional judgements) that result from them in an easily readable and understandable form for those interested, for example patients, their relatives and even lawyers.

Some fifteen or more years ago, a surgeon shared with us at a workshop we were running, his experience of sharing one of his reflections with a patient's family. Unexpectedly the patient had died following routine surgery. There was no case of negligence implied but there was, (understandably) considerable unhappiness and a growing hostility by the relatives leading up to a coroner's inquest. The surgeon, a wise and thoughtful person, wrote for himself a reflective account of what exactly had happened and how it had affected him. The surgeon told us that one day quite out of the blue he had the idea of sharing his own account of things with the relatives. This he did. The effect of this was quite profound. The relationship between the doctor and the relatives became much more open and communicative. The coroner's inquest went without incident and the case was closed. No one was more surprised by this than the senior surgeon.

We are of the opinion that what the relatives saw at first in this surgeon was what Osler in 1889, as quoted by Launer, 2019, described as *'The noble quality of imperturbability'*. The spontaneous act to share his reflection resulted, here, in a good outcome. Suddenly the family saw him as a human being and understood his thinking and the effect of this death on him as well as on themselves.

We explored in Chapter One the considerable dis-ease that is already well developed in the profession of medicine and some of the reasons for it. The growing gap between doctors and society needs thoughtful and disciplined attention (Blond et al., 2015) if the trust that vulnerable patients accord to us is to be maintained. The increasing emphasis on 'patient-centred care' needs doctors to consider and share the unmeasurable but highly significant elements of their practice more widely if the responsibilities of the doctor and the patient are to develop in harmony.

The appraiser and the doctor and vice versa

As we have already said in Chapter Four, in the UK, annual appraisal is a professional requirement for licenced medical practitioners. Reflective Practice is a requirement as part of this process. Our teaching of Reflective Practice and in particular written reflection, to many doctors, has been well received and has changed perceptions of what can be achieved *by doing it for the right reasons*.

We believe that Reflective Practice for doctors should be the central tenet of appraisal. Done well, it counterbalances the current focus of appraisal, which is mostly on the measurable elements of practice, by placing, at the centre of the process who the doctor is as a person, a professional practitioner and a servant of society. What a doctor is really doing here is researching their own practice in order to develop it with the aim of improving the quality of patient care.

How does this inform and justify plans for CPD?

All doctors need to make a case for how their continuing professional development is planned and structured. Using appropriate case narratives to show what you do and the breadth of their expertise will give sound evidence to support their arguments for CPD to continue to grow and mature as a senior doctor.

Responding to complications and complaints

The structure that we have offered through the TRP works extremely well as a framework for unpacking a doctor's actions and decision making in cases of complications and complaint. Used by each member of a clinical team in response to contentious cases, the process brings each member's own analysis and insights to case discussions and hugely empowers members to engage in the process and sharpen their thinking.

The Vital need for Researching Reflective Practice as a means of developing Medical Practice

As we look to the future however, we see a major need to ensure that this Transformative Reflective Process does not become just another protocol to be followed mindlessly. Rigorous research into better understanding the nuances and subtleties of medical practice through reflective writing and how this may be used for professional development needs urgent attention.

We have used, as an example of how such research may be focused, the GMCs requirements for Appraisal (see Table 4.11.1). Critique of the categories of the domains chosen by the GMC should also be part of this particular exploration. Such research would need good qualitative methodology to explore the underlying qualities of the doctor that lie beneath the visible tip of their performance and how these may be nurtured and developed. Research across all areas of where reflection is required in medical practice is vital but currently is shockingly absent.

Table 4.11.1 Ideas for informing research into TRP and Appraisal

Foci to inform research questions in all domains	GMC Domains For Appraisal	Foci to inform research questions in each domains
Where have these GMC domain categories (see the middle column) come from? Does the TRP writing illuminate more fully the qualitative evidence in the portfolio What has it highlighted and how? How did this inform the Appraisal Summary and Advice for future professional development? What was the nature of any surprises that emerged through Reflective Writing offered at Appraisal? Is there TRP evidence of professional development over a series of cases offered at appraisals? How do these four domains encourage exploration by appraiser and appraisee, of the qualities of wisdom, Professional Judgement, moral agency and professionalism of the doctor all of which are endemic to wise practice?	*Knowledge, Skills and Performance*	What knowledge used by the doctor is gleaned from the TRP writing that is not obvious in the quantitative data? How do the chosen domain of *Knowledge Skills and Performance* influence the format in which the information is offered? Is it more about numbers as data rather than the understanding of the doctor's new insights into their performance? Is the performance of the doctor that of a professional or only a technical worker? How does this domain heading invite flexible and imaginative thinking about what a doctor is and stands for?
	Safety and Quality	What does the TRP offer as a tried and tested way and a means of exploring the more humane qualities of the doctor? How does TRP help to tease out the quality (rather than the quantity of things done) of a doctor's attention to detail?
	Communications, Team work and Partnership	These are dependent on the kind of person the doctor is and how they see others. What is it that leads patients to trust doctors and vice versa?
	Maintaining Trust	What are the characteristics of the doctor/patient relationship that either maintains or destroys trust between doctors/ their patients and their relatives? What role do complications and unexpected consequences play in either maintaining or destroying trust between doctors/ their patients and their relatives?

Chapter Eleven

The implications for other professions beyond healthcare

This book has been focused on physicians and surgeons. We have considerable experience of working across many of the professions in healthcare but despite encouragement from those we have taught we have little experience of using these resources with professions *outside* healthcare. We do see however that at the level of principle they offer a potentially valuable resource to those who may be seeking to articulate more explicitly, the complexities of their professional practice.

The principles that The Transformative Reflective Process would offer to the wider professional community are listed below. The TRP offers *any* professional the following adapted list as a means of:

- improving their *detailed* understanding of their current practice and of themselves in that practice
- enabling their thinking and being to be unearthed, critiqued and developed
- providing a means of being far more articulate about their expertise
- enabling them to share this expertise far more broadly
- placing persuasive evidence on record of their regular exploration and refinement of their practice
- contributing to legal cases, crucial detailed information of a professional's judgements and of the custom and practice of their profession
- enabling society and individuals if shared more widely, to understand much better the complexity of a professional's decision making and their human and humane response to their professional responsibilities.

Attending to all of this, will, we believe, nurture self-knowledge, confidence and the recognition of the unmasterable capacity that is wisdom.

Endnote

Perhaps as professionals we should all seek to share our thinking and experience across professions and beyond them all. The caveat of course would be to maintain confidentiality and so speak at the level of principle. All of this requires research and refinement in order to ensure a freshness and relevance of the resource of TRP to professional development.

Chapter Twelve

Mind your heart! Considering spiritual perspectives in reviewing your chosen case

Della Fish, in conversation with Monica Butler RSM and Ann Hopper PhD

> Introduction
> Seeing with the heart not the head
> Aims and Intentions of this chapter
> The structure of this chapter
> Two key perspectives on wisdom
> A brief contextual survey of some ideas and values that challenge our understanding of spirituality
> A conversation exploring spiritual practice and spiritual wisdom
> The wisdom of the heart: an heuristic for a new Invisible.
> Endnote

Introduction

Whilst working with over 500 senior doctors in the NHS in the UK on Reflection for Medical Practice, we have come to understand more deeply the importance of a spiritual dimension in our professional lives, which profoundly influences our thinking and actions. We believe that spiritual ways of seeing and knowing already resonate with many professional practitioners, either tacitly or explicitly. Such a focus of understanding is becoming of interest within the professions more broadly and seems set to be even more significant in the third decade of the twenty-first century. This is particularly in the light of the pandemic of 2020 with all the uncertainty felt world-wide.

Certainly, it seems that people are suddenly realising that to do their job in the NHS, all practitioners have to hold deep-felt values which have for so long and persistently been denigrated and denied by those re-engineering the NHS. We believe that it is highly significant that Boris Johnson, the British Prime Minister spoke on Easter Sunday 2020, of the NHS as being 'the beating heart of this country.....It is powered by Love'. However, most professionals and many others are not always able to find the language and concepts through which to articulate spiritual matters and spiritual questions. Thus, this chapter will have a very different focus and flavour from those found in earlier parts of this book. It will offer language from other dimensions of human life, the spiritual, the poetic, the visionary and the mystical, which touch us all, whatever our explicit beliefs. It will offer readers of every persuasion or none, some ideas on how these enrich the understanding of the complexity of clinical practice and of being a clinical practitioner.

An example of this growing interest can also be found in Mahendran's recent work on how the individually unique and often unanticipated — and entirely unmeasurable and invisible — events of surgical practice will impact on our professional *beliefs* and may even reshape our thinking and how we see the world (Mahendran, 2019). Interestingly she grounds this idea in *haecceity*. This is a term from medieval scholastic philosophy and Christian spirituality, first emerging through the Franciscan followers of Duns Scotus (c. 1266 – 1308), and used to name the discrete qualities, properties or characteristics of a thing that make it a *particular* thing. *Haecceity* is a person's or an object's *thisness*. This idea was taken up by the nineteenth century Jesuit Priest and poet Gerard Manley Hopkins (Urban, 2018), who felt that everything in the universe was characterised by what he called inscape, the distinctive design that constitutes individual identity. This identity is not static but dynamic, and it is far from, and much deeper than what those in the professions are used to referring to as 'professional identity'. It sees each 'being' in the universe as enacting its own unique identity. And the human being, the most individually distinctive being in the universe, recognises the inscape of other beings and thus sees the world in greater wonder. But, significantly, the seeing is carried out by the heart, not the head.

Seeing with the heart not the head

Whilst this is a problematic notion at one level and not always easy to grasp, it has a quality of common understanding about it. For example, we all are familiar with the idea 'I knew in my heart this was not going to work!'. The underlying point that this makes, is that the speaker has had an instinctive sense from viewing the activity step by step and also in retrospect as a whole, that despite other positive indicators there was an overall feeling that not everything fitted. This scrutinising, both step by step and as a retrospective overview, carried out in a meticulous and disciplined manner, as we have described in the earlier chapters of this book, will help us understand better the influence of the unmeasurable elements of practice. We would argue that the significance of such exploration relies more on the quality of this review than on the length of time spent on it. The practical implications of this are pursued in the final section of this chapter.

Aims and Intentions of this Chapter

Our broad aim then in this chapter is to help to fuel the spiritual energy and ideas of all professionals who work on the ground to tackle the problems of our time, and to serve the public and nurture humanity with 'a good' (like education, justice, and health). Our central intention is to encourage professionals to explore ways of articulating the nature of their own spiritual understanding and how this relates to their daily practice. I, (Della Fish) do not have the expertise to articulate and offer such enlightenment, but by listening to and sharing the conversation of two life-long practitioners of differing but similar belief-driven spiritual practice (Christianity), I try to make it possible here to articulate and examine the spiritual wisdom common to those of faith or no faith that can more consciously guide how we live. Thus we are using the term spiritual in this chapter to indicate a distinction between religious beliefs which are individual to us, and a sense of the spiritual where anyone may feel humility about their place in the universe. This chapter also seeks to provide a framework and language with which to articulate, share and explore elements of spirituality in practice.

Our intentions here then, are to sketch ways in which spiritual perspectives in our lives can bring us to recognise what we are coming to call *The wisdom of the Heart*, and which we offer at the end of this chapter as another potential Invisible. We all experience such perspectives in some way or another, quite *irrespective* of details about our religion, faith or no faith, and our background and culture. So, for example, our 'being' and our values are probably driven in some way by the way our heart shapes how we see ourselves and the world, and how far we let awe at the world we live and work in, influence our personhood, our conduct, our decisions and our relationships. Further, our 'knowing' does not all come from the mind. We drew attention to the phrase "I knew in my heart that x would happen". Some would of course say that is 'intuition' and subscribe to psychological ways of articulating this which try to make it less abstract, and even render it 'measurable'. But equally, from a more centrally spiritual perspective, writers have seen and explored this as 'The discernment of the Heart', or as Joycelin Dawes characterises it *Discernment and Inner Knowing*. (Dawes, 2017).

We noted with interest in Her Majesty The Queen's Easter speech of 2020 that she saw the current pandemic 'as opportunity to slow down, pause and reflect in prayer or meditation'. We also noted the echo of our comments above in her speech when she said of voluntary isolation: "we know, deep down, that it is the right thing to do".

In this chapter therefore we seek to share ideas about spiritual wisdom that might enrich and even transform *any* practitioner's understanding of the depth of their own being, whatever other informing and underlying theories influence the way they seek to practice. Thus, we are exploring spiritual wisdom itself, and how it might be understood and drive the understandings and practices of those in medicine, healthcare and other professions. So, this chapter is about our own 'Being, Knowing, Doing, Thinking, and Becoming as professionals', not about how to respond to the spiritual needs of patients, as for example offered by Cobb et al., 2012; Gordon et al., 2011; Rogers and Wattis, 2015, and Wattis et al., 2017.

We also offer further perspectives on *The Invisibles*, which, as we reach for the future will need even greater exploration. In much – but not all – of what we have previously written, we have used our minds to explore and characterise the Being, Knowing, Doing, Thinking and Becoming, that we argue constitute the core of wise professional practice, and to characterise some categories of invisible influences on professional practice that we are not always conscious of without reflection on our own work.

Thus, although much of this book is about Aristotle's practical reasoning and his views on professional judgement, we are not promoting here a dualistic alternative choice between Aristotle's ideas and those emanating from spiritual wisdom, as if one or the other holds the golden key to wise practice. Rather, we suggest that they should be used together. We live in a coloured world and try to see the wholeness of life even when it *appears* to be only either black or white (both of which of course contain all colours even though we don't see them). That is why we also aspire to encourage deliberation (which seeks to find a more wholistic way forward that offers the best for all) rather than debate (which seeks to polarise ideas into acceptable or not acceptable).

The structure of this chapter

The rest of this chapter contains four related sections. Firstly, offered briefly, are some key definitions and significant characteristics of two differing perspectives on wisdom within professional practice. We see as found *both* in Aristotle's views about wise practical reasoning, (see *Nicomachean Ethics* which lies behind several of our original Invisibles) and also our understanding about spiritual wisdom as drawn from the *Perennial Tradition* (Huxley, 1945) and ideas about Spiritual Discernment of the heart (Dawes, 2017). We do not claim that these are the only ways of seeing wisdom in practice, but wonder if they might represent positions on a spectrum of ideas about wisdom that practitioners of all faiths and none might need to explore in the future.

The next section sets the context for the ensuing conversation, by highlighting briefly, as a background to Section Three, some challenging aspects of 21st century life that make the work of professionals even more demanding today than in earlier times. This leads into Section Three which is the centre of what we offer. The content here emerges mainly through a conversation between two Christian professionals, which seeks to capture ways of articulating some of the essence of spiritual wisdom in practice. It offers deep insights into spiritual understanding and practice that are valuable for all practitioners. It may need several readings and exploration to glean these insights.

The chapter ends with the fourth and final section, in which we introduce a new heuristic that represents the *Invisibles of the Heart* and we speculate on ways in which some new prompts might enrich further the processes of transformative reflection on practice.

Two key perspectives on wisdom

Aristotle's ideas about wisdom in practice

The popularity of Aristotle's ideas about practical reasoning in the West in the last forty years has seen most professional practitioners influenced by neo-Aristotelian versions of wisdom and practical reasoning, as characterised by *phronesis* and *praxis*. For Aristotle, wisdom was the highest virtue. Fish (2012: prelims) offers a definition of ideas found in his *Nicomachean Ethics*, as follows.

Phronesis is the disposition to act wisely or prudently in a specific situation. Its aim is to do what is morally right and proper in that situation. The action (*Praxis*) which it engages in is morally committed action, in which and through which our values are given practical expression. The forms of thinking it brings to practice include clinical reasoning, deliberation, and professional judgement.

Schwartz and Sharpe (2011) remind us that there appears to be a broad consensus that such wisdom is associated with a long list of virtues which are practised for their own sake. For Aristotle, such virtues drive our decisions and actions and are to be found in the mean or average point between two extremes.

MacIntyre (1981/2007) however, argues that: 'there are in our present society a number of rival and incompatible accounts of virtues', and that 'ours is a society lacking a shared morality' such that the 'possibilities of shared moral education are not what they are sometime taken to be'. Further, not every idea can readily be properly translated from Aristotle's ancient context to our modern world.

Aristotle's ideas about practical wisdom have however, been taken up on a large scale in professional practice, and his concepts and language have enabled practitioners to gain a better understanding of their own conduct and decision making through reflective explorations (both oral and written). (See de Cossart and Fish, 2005; Fish and de Cossart, 2007 and 2013.) Such reflective approaches owe something at least to the seminal work of Schön (1978), and to a considerable number of books and papers on both reflection and practical (or 'clinical') reasoning, that have been generated within many professions (see for example the fifth edition of one seminal text: Higgs, et al., 2018, and also Boniface and Fish, 2012).

Spiritual wisdom: starting points

A very different but not incompatible way of conceiving of practice wisdom is revealed by exploring *spiritual* wisdom and its practices. Here, wisdom is seen to arise from the heart which is seen as discerning truth more accurately than can the mind alone. 'The heart' here is used to mean far more than our shared modern idea that the heart is simply the centre of emotion, but rather that it is the fount of love which discerns the best way forward for us and those we care for (professionally as well as personally).

Spirituality is problematic to define, and indeed some practitioners much prefer to substitute for 'define' the less dualistic term 'describe', which is why this section is called 'starting points'. Perhaps the word 'spirituality' stands for the way we search for meaning and seek to live out our fundamental beliefs and values in everyday life. In Christian terms, spirituality refers to the way our fundamental beliefs, values and practices reflect our understanding of and relationship with God. Some would argue for something like our own attempt at a definition, as follows.

> The word 'spirituality' in most contexts indicates the way that, in seeking to live out our deepest and most fundamental beliefs and values, we are searching for meaning.

This would mean for those who subscribe to most faiths, spirituality refers to the way our fundamental beliefs, values and practices reflect our understanding of and relationship with God (however we might characterise God). For those who are of no faith it nonetheless can bring a re-recognition of our place in the world and a reminder of some ideas we probably once dismissed. This would indicate a sense of something larger, beyond our own small world, that is in some way sacred and which suggests the need to seek the source of our inner being.

Following this, in essence then, spiritual understanding seems to be about 'coming home to oneself' – recognising and thus being able to use in practice the resources gifted to us, *that we all already have within us*. Everything else flows from this, and as Huxley (1945) points out most spiritual ideas and actions sprang originally from man's early beliefs in powers beyond us.

This way of seeing is agreed by many as rooted in an ancient tradition of ideas from the Perennial Tradition, a continuous stream that dates back to antiquity and has surfaced from time to time through the Middle Ages to the present, in the West, where it was highlighted by, for example, people like the unknown author of the Middle English treatise *The Cloud of Unknowing*; Hildegard of Bingen (1098 – 1117); Mechtilde of Magdaburg (1210 – 1282); Meister Eckhart (1260 -1328) , Julianna of Norwich (1342 -1416), and more recently Thomas Merton (1915 – 1968), Thomas Keating (1923 - 2012), Richard Rohr (1943 -), Cynthia Bourgeault (1947-) and Echart Tolle (1948 -).

Aldous Huxley said that: 'rudiments of the perennial philosophy may be found among the traditional lore of primitive peoples in every region of the world, and in its fully developed forms it has a place in every one of the higher religions' (Huxley, 1945 vii). At the heart of perennial philosophy is 'the wager' that there is a common spiritual ground that is shared by the many religions of the world. Perennial philosophy is the (sometimes forgotten) backbone of what are called the "spiritual but not religious," and "new-age" philosophies. Simultaneously, it is one of the most inspiring and widespread influences in modern spirituality and also one of the most fervently critiqued approaches to religious pluralism and interreligious dialogue.

Some say that the Perennial Philosophy is in some ways the ruling spiritual philosophy of our time, including in its ranks everyone from Sam Harris to Abraham Maslow to Ken Wilber and to HRH Prince Charles. It is perhaps interesting that the future defender of the Anglican faith in the UK is a devotee of Perennialism (see *The Sacred Web: A Journal of Tradition and Modernity*: Sept 23rd - 24th 2006). http://www.sacredweb.com/conference06/conference_introduction.html

The discernment of the heart

A further component of this whole spiritual perspective is offered by the Quaker author Dawes (2017) who argues that making decisions for the best, rests in calling on discernment [of the heart] which is about 'inner knowing'. Dawes sums this up by arguing that:

> What is clear is that discernment embraces a considered way of deciding that is resonant with our deepest values and calls forth action guided by wisdom, compassion, love and truth. Some may call this God and others express it in a variety of ways.
> (Dawes, 2017: 78.)

Practical reasoning and the wisdom of the heart

We would see possibilities in bringing together the practical reasoning of Aristotle and Spiritual wisdom which we now call the wisdom of the heart. Practical reasoning attends to the understandings of the mind and might be complemented by being followed and checked out by the discernment of the heart. (See the final section of this chapter.)

Spiritual wisdom, then, is not about following set guidelines, but about 'being'. It stems from awareness of the spiritual (even the divine) in us, and gaining a deeper understanding of our true nature and its relationship to that 'Source beyond us' that fuels our being and actions, which some will call God and some will see as mysterious.

Thus, spiritual wisdom is not the gathering of more facts and information, as if that would coalesce into truth. On the contrary, it is closer to home. To engage in spiritual thought and discourse is not to play with complex and abstract philosophical ideas nor to enter into an impersonal world of 'proof and truth'. Rather, as Carr says, spiritual discourse:

> serves a logical and practical purpose in our lives [and is] rather different from the language of scientific exploration. It is primarily concerned not to identify facts or truths but to express attitudes, values or commitments. It is about making more explicit a personal vision of our relationship to that which endures forever.
> (Carr, D., 2002:151.)

This demands of us 'a growing awareness of, and sensitivity to how we conceive of life, and a commitment to our kinship with and responsibilities to, humanity and the world in which we live'. Carr continues by saying that: 'Such developing levels of understanding open up new concepts that language previously has seemed to pin down too simplistically'. Such a sense of that vision can only be expressed in 'a language of spirit and soul' as is often found in metaphor and poetry, (Carr, D., 2002: 500).

So, this is about seeing, knowing and being in a new way that is perhaps truer to our whole selves. It is about heart as well as mind. Further, a spiritually grounded practitioner will seek to go beyond the dividing and reductionist boundaries of the current dualities endemic in today's western culture, and thus gain a more peaceable and less anxious existence. Thus, we are trying to explore bringing together Aristotle's wisdom of the mind, and spiritual understanding of the importance of the wisdom of the heart.

Clearly, spirituality is likely to need the strengthening support from our sense of what Carr calls 'the Source beyond us', which will be interpreted differently by different people, but which inevitably assumes some form of private appreciative monologue, prayer or meditation, often found in what Rohr calls 'sacred silence' which is larger than simply a lack of audible noise, but which happens when thought becomes its own kind of fullness with its own kind of sweet voice. (Daily Meditation from the Centre for Action and Contemplation, 09.01.20. See also: cac.org: Contemplative appendix to the Daily Meditations).

Of course, there is no standard model of meditation. So, for example, it is important to note that the 'inner contemplative tradition' is not the same as Mindfulness (which has become a major business enterprise in the USA). Mindfulness focuses on what is going on inside and outside ourselves, moment by moment whereas contemplative or centering prayer (Keating, 2001) is seen by some as the mainstay of spiritual practice. It 'puts the mind in the heart' [defined as the centre of wisdom and therefore of discernment] and strives for 'objectless awareness' which enables a new form of perception of the unity of the whole world made by a cosmic creator whose home is already in our hearts. This requires, as Bourgeault (2016) suggests, a whole new 'operating system' in our minds and hearts. It is not just coming from a new version of perception that is still actually embedded in previous ways of seeing, and which still focuses on the presumed 'duality in everything'.

Since any 'practice' inevitably operates from within a given practice, or at least makes close reference to the traditions of that practice, so spiritual practice can be fully realised only in the presence of a spiritual tradition' (Horujy, 2015: 118). It is a shared human journey. But some of its concepts and therefore language could be used by practitioners and other workers, within their reflections on and explorations of their practice. We would say that as part of developing Reflective Practice, individuals need to explore their own understanding of spirituality.

Through the conversation offered below in Section Three, we try to illustrate how, for professional practitioners, awareness of our inner resources can help us to recognise and honour those deep aspects of our being that we can bring to the service of others, and which, once recognised, can provide a well-spring of strong resilience and persistence in difficult times, and deep joy and fulfilment in better moments. First, however we offer a brief survey or reminder of some contextual issues that form the background to our conversation.

A brief contextual survey of some ideas and values that challenge our understanding of spirituality

In this section, we acknowledge what seem to be some key challenges that form a context for and a stark contrast to the following conversation. Such challenges shape decisions about practice and are faced by professionals, often on a daily basis. They arise from the dire state of the current Western world in which we work and live, and highlight its current broken character, however we also highlight that some writers are more positive about how we might see these issues differently and conduct ourselves accordingly by considering the supreme purposes of our life and work.

The current character of our broken society, its dehumanised values and how we might respond

There is clearly a pervasive sense within our society, not only in the UK but in much of the world, that something is wrong with western culture in our current attitudes, values, assumptions and beliefs and thus the actions and reactions they lead to. This is most strongly highlighted in the context of public-service professions that affect us all, like Healthcare, Education and the Law. Here, it is glaringly obvious that practitioners regard their working context as in such a dire state that the quality of their work (once seen as service to humanity), and thus their pride in it, have been almost totally eroded so that their patients, students and clients no longer have much trust in the system. Striking descriptions of the problems and possible responses are briefly offered from the writings, of for example of Bauman, 2000; Wilkinson and Pickett, 2010; Welby, 2016 and 2018; and Hordern, 2018.

Bauman, 2000, offered us the memorable metaphor 'Liquid Modernity' to capture the excessive flexibility that is beyond 'fluidity', which is required of us all by obsessive modernization (sic) and the consequent 'unstoppable rising volume of "uprooted" people'. He warned us of the disappearance of the solid structures and institutions that once provided the stable foundations for well-ordered modern societies, and of the consequences for individuals and communities. His memorable phrase that captures the negative energy of all this is: 'When elephants fight, pity the grass' (Oxford Dictionary of Proverbs). Quoting Alain Peyrefitte (1998) and the works of Bourdieu, Bauman highlights the most prominent characteristic of this society as false confidence —in self, in others and in institutions, all of which sustain each other unquestioningly. In response, Bauman argued for a version of communitarianism and its respect for and need to uphold society's moral character.

In similar vein, Wilkinson and Pickett (2010) who, perhaps following Mary Douglas's (1986) much earlier protest about the 'inhumanity of institutions', highlighted in *The Spirit Level* the evidence that 'we have got close to the end of what economic growth can do for us', and the cost of it in the loss of welfare and happiness (p.5). Their way forward is to 'map out ways in which the new society can begin to grow within and alongside institutions' and gradually marginalise and replace them, (Wilkinson and Pickett, 2010: 236).

One might argue that the above possible ways forward do not conceive of whole new ways of seeing and acting and thus are not truly transformational and are devoid of any explicitly shared view of the specific foundational human, moral and spiritual values upon which any serious change would need to be based. Thus, they do not contain any 'soul-food', which in a startling metaphor, perhaps aptly captures the spiritual aridity of the proposed solutions and their lack of any nourishing energy.

By contrast we might begin with the notion that: 'Our supreme purpose in this life is not to make a fortune, nor to pursue pleasure, nor to write our name on history but to discover the spark of the Divine that is in our hearts', (see Easwaran, (1996). Thus, the more recent work of, for example, Welby (2016 and 2018) and Hordern (2018) start in a different place that is both more optimistic and more grounded in the whole person we are, such that we can begin, in the words of Welby's book title, to engage in 'Dethroning Mammon' (Welby, 2016).

He argues that the marketisation of healthcare in the UK has led to mammon's consequent mastery of its relationships, and the idea that our ability to spend validates our personhood. Here, the culture of the 'Bottom Line', has invaded healthcare and devalued all that more spiritual understanding that many are wanting to bring to the surface. Perhaps more insidiously it has devalued people with life-limiting illnesses and those whose autonomy is threatened by handicaps of all kinds. Thus, Mammon offers us economics that rest on the implication that we only value what we measure. This results in us ignoring the voluntary and un-remunerated work, thus 'demean[ing] those who act from love' (Welby, 2016: 14 and 15 - 18). All this prevents us from seeing differently, and recognising that 'what is not measurable may be valuable beyond measure' (Welby, 2016: 40). He argues that only through individuals who transform their seeing, listening, and understanding, can a different world begin to emerge. Taking this further in his most recent book, he places the responsibility for "reimagining Britain", and the creating of a new narrative of hope, on the intermediate institutions of family, education, health, housing and economics, such that key moral values are reinstituted within our practices (Welby, 2018).

Hordern focuses on the destruction that has accompanied the standardised hyper-efficient processes that have 'robbed healthcare professionals of a patient, conscientious compassionate, joyful and authoritative sense of vocation.' He says that 'determining what *mastery* and *service* mean is central to any ethically and culturally sophisticated interpretation of marketisation's multiple influences amidst the suffering which healthcare is instituted to address'. His response to the 'commodification of care' and the 'distortion of compassion' is to strive for a new covenant (rather than contract) between government, representing society, and those who serve individuals who are part of the public, in which both are bound to one another not by transactions of power or wealth, but by '*hessed*', (covenant love, expressed in deeds). He offers a range of issues which ought to be attended to within such covenants.

These concerns and possible solutions offer a backdrop against which individual practitioners have to work. But they do not show them why and how practice wisdom can transform people and their practices for the common good. The following conversation therefore offers a flavour of spiritual practice, its wisdom and what it can achieve. It will benefit most those who having read it, then re-read it, when best insights will be gained.

Chapter Twelve

A conversation exploring spiritual practice and spiritual wisdom

The interaction that follows is between **MB**, Sister Monica Butler and **AH**, Dr Ann Hopper, who have each worked in very different professional practices and come from different spiritual traditions, but who share fundamentally Christian values, and beliefs. **DF**, Della Fish was merely a facilitator and writer up of the agreed resulting understandings that emerged.

For the sake of succinctness and logic, we present here an edited version, agreed between the three of us, of what were two recorded, free-ranging and unrehearsed conversations between MB and AH. In each they shared ideas about their attempts in practice to live the spiritual life and focused on trying to clarify the key tenets of spiritual wisdom that underlie their thought and action. Each recording was over an hour long and they were about three weeks apar. They were firstly fully transcribed, and then scrutinised, corrected and critiqued by the participants. A very few simple oral transcription symbols were used, because our interest was solely in the content and ideas not with detailed Conversation Analysis (See for example, Hutchby and Wooffitt, (1999). Thus, the thoughtfulness of speakers, in the struggle to articulate ideas as precisely as possible, is shown by dots, and en-lines are used when the spoken sentence became more complex. Only full utterances were numbered. Occasionally, as in most talk, some utterances are not full sentences.

The conversation

> 1.DF: So Sister Monica, Dr Ann Hopper, thank you for being willing to try to articulate some complex and difficult ideas, that might help us find new ways of being, seeing, and thinking about spirituality, and particularly spiritual wisdom in action. Could you begin by telling us something about yourselves, … Sister Monica?
>
> 2. MB: Yes. I am a Sister of Mercy, which effectively means I am what is commonly called a nun. I am an active sister, working out among people in the streets and homes of East London, not in an institution at all. But I belong to a religious order that seeks to live a simple and a spiritual life, so I am constantly reminded in my own commitment to the way of life – of the dimension which is always below the surface of everything I do, which animates me, comforts me, and which encourages me, but which is very difficult to describe.
>
> By background and training I am a secondary teacher and worked in an industrial city in the North of England with youngsters who were beautifully honest and truthful but who did not find the factual teaching that I was offering them very satisfying. Often at the end of a class two or three boys and girls would come up to the desk when everyone else had left the room and ask me a question which exposed a level of both vulnerability and interest, but when I said: "OK this is great, can we look at this in the next lesson?". They did not want the class to know they had asked.
>
> Faced with this vulnerability when exploring inner concepts, visions and feelings, except in a safe environment, I changed my tactics and I began to explore contexts in which

youngsters could look below the surface of their life — at their values, decisions —to discover their own meaning. They were very responsive, as years later were adults who also grappled with the same issues — how to explore their inner world, discover who they truly were and gain the confidence to be authentic, and then express that in the world, in their relationships, in their work. So, using the Socratic method of not telling but raising their interests with a question, gradually I began to understand that people learn best if they have the opportunity to make their own inner journey into this rather dark and mysterious place within, where there is so much untapped wisdom. They need to come, for themselves, to their truth, their knowing, their true self, to their level of compassion, which is deep and meaningful.

4. AH: I think I grew up in a place where authority was always outside oneself —in a conventional English Christian family — and was taught to look to the Scriptures and the church for moral authority and ways of living. And that sense of authority was reinforced —in the Fifties anyway — by student nurse training, and midwifery training, both through the people who were responsible for us and the textbooks we studied. And it wasn't until much later, when I took the educational adventure of thinking and reading with the help of a very good supervisor, that I began to see that in learning, particularly in health care, having no answer is not the same as having no response … that in many ways responses may be more profound than answers.

So how does that work out now, at the other end of my life? I try to live this within my work in a hospital Chaplaincy. It has to be said that hospitals are places in which I feel very much at home. I have nursed in them, delivered babies and taught in them, been a patient in one, um but … and it's a big but … coming, as it were with none of my old professional expertise to offer, with nothing to offer from the point of view of the authorities and old certainties with which I grew up, all I had was a human response to human suffering. And the best place it seemed for me to work out that sense and do something with it was in a hospital Chaplaincy. The team, which is very broad, not only interdenominational but interfaith, opened my eyes to what we all had in common, which was a sense of our common humanity when faced with the difficulty of those things which we cannot understand and for which no one simple authority will give us an answer.

So, I had to move from the certainties of Christianity to the mysteries which the Mystics took, as it were, for granted, and try to live without that external authority but with some deep sense that the occasional brief momentary, fragments of insight which I gleaned from the Mystics. They became what I wanted to live by, and I found it was, in some very profound sense, already there inside me, if only I could access it. So, there was some way in which I needed the inner and the outer to become one and not two separate things.

Does anything in what I have just said resonate with anything that you would want to reinforce, or say more clearly than I do, Sister Monica?

5. MB: Well, I want to *engage* with it … you mention the Mystics and we have given indicators that we shall mention them and have given brief details earlier in this chapter, but for some readers, I imagine, that would be out of their experience.

6. AH: So for me it is about the resources that become available from the mystery of the whole person deep within ourselves... that they ultimately come from the mystery of the whole universe or God, and that understanding comes from the Perennial Philosophy.

7. MB: Here, the 'inner path of life', unique as it is to each individual, reaches towards a realm beyond materialism, a sphere where things matter beyond that which can be touched, acquired, measured or seen, and which we call spiritual. And then comes the tricky part, which is trusting in one's own experience as one's principal teacher, and 'winnowing your experience of life to beget wisdom' (Rohr), which is far from looking for top-down doctrine to obey, but rather beginning from the bottom up by acting in alignment with all that one understands of truth and love, and reflecting on what happens. Thus, faith is not so much something we 'have' as something we attempt to live by, meeting life with love rather than anxiety, and sustaining that with contemplative silence, both alone and in a worshipping group

In my case, not being sure I had done my pupils any service, because I had alerted them to something that somehow they couldn't take anywhere, I turned to working with adults because their resources are more plentiful, and the mystics provide much of this. I encourage them to try to understand mysticism, because that is where each person is called to go — that is, to be a mystic. And ...um ... I think this chapter is moving towards um alerting people to the fact that they can access these things and where they can go for this.

8. AH: Well, I found that too. In reading at his request, from the work of Meister Eckhart, to a blind scholar, I came to recognise that — just as responses are more important than answers, so mystery wasn't something *to find an answer for*, but to enjoy, accept, rest into and live alongside. I can only call it relaxing into a sense that mystery wasn't something to be feared but engaged with in some sort of safety.

9. MB: I'm wondering: are we stumbling upon the heart of this chapter, that ...that secret ... that either enables or prevents us from being good practitioners in whatever we do? Because we do seem to have a sense that anything that is mysterious, is unknowable, far away ...even an illusion, but it's not.

So, there is a difference between having the facts and being told what to do, and seeing rather that it's more about my response to the facts and the experience — and that's where we begin to appreciate enlightenment, inner being, inner knowing, inner authority. And we actually experience it *in the event* in which we are engaged... That's what I think is at the heart of Mysticism. It's not about facts and belief systems. Its ..

{10. AH: [interrupts] .... it's about being at home without them!

11. MB: Hmmm. That's lovely because that points us back to the sense of belonging to the things that we are doing. We are not strangers, handling information, handing facts, handling material, we are engaging with what those facts and relationships etc are about ... And that is: to help this person to greater wholeness, integration, inner strength, whatever it is, we are engaging in *praxis*.... There is something magic or you could say mystical when we engage with another person at the level of the heart and we somehow convey a sense of respect, of faith in them, of even love... that person never forgets and

that's I think the root [of the spiritual dimension] we are trying to explore. How do you access the spiritual dimension that is deep in the heart of all human experience? In fact, I would go so far as to say of every aspect of Creation. There is something mystical, something communicating its life to the rest of *us*.

Thus, we enable both ourselves and the other to begin to recognise the mysterious elements that most of us keep hidden or don't even kind of surface in consciousness. If somebody else engages us at that level, it almost wakens it up. So, I am wondering: Do we, as professionals, have the capacity to be at the level of awareness with each person we are privileged to serve and to awaken in them the response (your word Ann). So that beyond engaging with the technical matters of our practice, we somehow engage with their inner self and our inner self, which knows the truth.

So, in returning to my true self, that is the essence of who I am at the depths of my being, I come to know that all I need is already within. I just have to realise it, "make it real", learn to enact it in everyday life. There is infinite resource within, and with practice I can access this wisdom more and more. Then there is a quiet confidence that arises in us when we are sufficiently aware of self, that translates into an authority and knowing. The word confidence comes from *con-fidere* (with strength) and so there is a confidence which is quite unconscious when I am in touch with my true self. Only when I have had the experience do I have the chance of getting the meaning. So much of this lies in our capacity to relate to others. I do it with the eye … and a stream of energy passes between us…

12. AH: … And I want to call it love.

13. MB: Yes! And of course. … and Richard Rohr says that kind of love is in the silent acceptance of the situation — which some people refer to as contemplation. When I focus my energies and attention on the goodness of the other … that some of us refer to as God … then I have the experience of that cycle of giving as also receiving. Rohr describes it as: 'closing the circle', which is a lovely idea, and makes a lot of sense…. It makes the whole thing generative.

For me, in my own ministry, working now with adults, and with groups who are not satisfied necessarily with their project or their outcomes… (so I work as a facilitator among them),….. it always has to be that in preparing for that work: I ask what is good for this group? And I don't know it, so I have to go in ignorant, and then discover it. It has to be found in them and their desire. And that would be the same in any individual work that seeks to vitalise, in a way, someone's inner life, inner authority, inner knowing.

I bring to it that aspect of myself (the heart) which allows me to discern the truth and, where I bring whatever I am learning, feeling, sensing and intuiting, I have a sense that this is 'that which I have known always' ..This knowledge that arises deep within self and can be filtered via head and mind is (in the Christian tradition) the kind of knowledge which 'wells up into eternal life'. We get excited because we know it! So, it is the heart that is the true seat of wisdom. But the Wisdom or Perennial Tradition is not about a club or rules … structures are not the essence of what we are about. Religion can be described as man's search for god and is a human construct. But the wisdom tradition presumes or indicates our true nature, which is already in the light and is divine. The implications of this are enormous, but the invitation to live from this truth must be the most attractive truth of all! And that is when we gawp ... and enter the silence — the otherness of ourselves ... The silence invites you into it... So if I can recognise the draining that is happening to me, and hang on [in quiet contemplation], I will be refreshed. Does that make sense to you?

14. AH: It makes perfect sense to me because, in the Chaplaincy work I do, some of it is what I call in a horrible phrase, "cold calling": walking up to a bed knowing absolutely nothing whatsoever about this person, having rapidly to establish some ... hopefully ... useful rapport with them, so that that response which you've so wonderfully described becomes a part of the encounter, so that ... not only do I begin to understand better where they may be coming from, but they also begin to understand better where I am at, and the relationship in some way becomes reciprocal. For me, every human encounter is significant, it's about what can be created in that moment to moment, human being to human being. It's about the vulnerability of us both. And it's costly... I feel the strength go out of me — and it's at that point that you can actually feel that some sort of human interaction can be meaningful — *and not without it!*

15. DF: So, how do you access and sustain that energy, when times are tough? Or do you never see them as tough? I struggle with being able to see the positive opportunities in everything that seems to be negative when I am trying to do some of the things that you talk about in a less experienced way than you both. Did Cynthia Bourgeault, (2016) capture it when she said you have to engage in a different 'operating system' — as in a computer that does different things from previously, not from a gradual degree of upgrade, but through a major almost technical transformation that sets things out quite differently and requires us to use quite different processes.

16: MB: Is it to do with a different level of self-knowledge that we have maybe come to, and are constantly developing, which enables us then to be truthful and to draw on our own resources more readily? If I am always trying to hide behind my persona, if I am always trying to present to you the nice front, if am so concerned with my appearance, I am not really going to be able to notice your need or your level of vulnerability. And I think what the mystics have offered us, and what the mystical life within each person is holding, is a level of resource and a level of gift and sensitivity and generosity and compassion, which is infinite, which is connected to the entire Universe, which puts me in a completely different, — you suggested 'operating system', Della — and that is what is so attractive, because it is so open and so fluid — but it's hands off.

17. AH: Its letting that be, and not fussing it and thinking that you have got to have completed it and that there has to be some conclusion that is identifiable. That interaction is a tiny, tiny, miniscule part of something hugely bigger than the encounter.

18. MB: So for example, in the accompaniment that I am involved in with individuals (as a Spiritual Director), I often have the experience of being with somebody for the 50 minutes we have contracted, and then as they go out, they say how much I have helped them, when I have hardly opened my mouth. Now to me that's a mystical encounter, and the doctor, teacher, practitioner of any kind, can, with some level of awareness, enter that and facilitate that in their own work. And it is not exhausting. In fact, it is almost

the opposite — exhilarating.

19. DF. But you are both practitioners of this way of living. Has it taken you a period of time to come to where you are now and what are the key moments that have helped you in that?

20. AH. For me it isn't more than the last 10 years ... But I want to be able to say, "No!". This mystery is available here and now and it isn't something to be worked on. It's to be accepted, appreciated, it isn't something you work at but something you acknowledge and accept, and glory in, almost.

It used to worry me, but now it's a sense that life is a great big woven tapestry, in which you might just pick up a dropped stitch and it might be nothing more significant than that but I just don't think.. um .. love is ever wasted or destroyed — and I just want to be part of that cycle.

{21. MB: I think we *were* much more relaxed about being in that cycle, when we were {children...

{AH: [softly] exactly

{MB: and we lose it and it becomes sophisticated and independent and I think possibly we're returning to it, learning 'to grow old gracefully' by getting more in touch with that constancy of loving within ourselves. But do you think in terms of practice, maybe this only comes to us in our senior years when we are really at ease with our practice?

22. AH ... And with the disconnectedness and unfinished nature — or apparent disconnectedness and unfinished nature of it (MB: Mmmm). It's what the new Chaplaincy Ward Visitors find hard — that there aren't conclusions, ... they want to be able to do something, to be able to come away feeling that something has been concluded, or some important transaction has occurred. I think you have to just not be concerned by that ... to recognise it and let it go.

23. MB: There's another question that you have offered us perhaps, Ann: How does this affect the way that we stand in front of others? Much of the concern of any medical practitioner would be, yes, the desire to alleviate suffering and illness, but, both in Chaplaincy work and in accompanying other people as I do, or actually being involved in medical practice, how does that affect the resources I bring to being with another in their suffering? What is it I am drawing on, or accessing or offering to the other in that context? And I suppose that one of the things I have been noticing in recent years — and I am like you Ann, I've come to much of this towards the end of my life, is that the point of the Christian practice and the understanding of the meaning of suffering is that it stops with me.... In the sense that I listen, and receive and know much of the suffering of the world, but in no way am I going to pass it on and punch your nose because I am upset by world events. ...I don't take this on and pass it on, extend it, multiply it, but it stops here.... which I think is the essence of what Jesus was doing in his life, death and resurrection. It stopped with him.

Chapter Twelve

So, does any practitioner actually have to be present to the one who is suffering or learning in such a way that they don't get all that confusion going on between the energies of that person and them. Do I stay clear, honest, true to myself and just simply radiate love?....

24. DF: Those last words seem a good place to stop. I can't thank you both enough for offering us a serious glimpse into your hearts and minds and of how you live your life. I think you have enriched what we can do by reflecting on the mystery of who we are.

The wisdom of the heart: an Heuristic for a new Invisible

All that we have offered in this chapter has driven us to begin to explore what kind of Invisible we might offer physicians and surgeons (if not also other professionals) to help them 'check out' whether the two exploratory Invisibles we have associated with Aristotle's practical reasoning also resonate with the wisdom of the heart.

Figure 4.12.1 The new heuristic: The wisdom of the heart

We have chosen in Figure 12.4.1, to represent a heuristic of 'putting the mind into the heart' by offering a heart with a sketch of the brain within it. This is a reminder that this new Invisible might be used both to clarify each of the Invisibles and also last of all, to check out that all the elements of the patient case fit together and are indeed compatible with whatever we might mean by spiritual wisdom. Please note: this will require you, in whatever time and place you can allow, to stand back from your chosen case, in what we have earlier learnt to call sacred silence, and consider the following prompts:

To clarify each of the Invisibles

- Have I just used measurable markers in considering this case or have I taken account of what I felt in my heart?
- Does all that I have done resonate with my most fundamental values and my whole 'being'?

To check out how the overall view of the case resonates with 'The wisdom of the heart'

- Does all that I have said, written, done and decided, resonate with my Inner Knowing?
- What kind of example from my own practice is *this* case?
- How have I dealt with the temptations to seek any possible false closure or a straightforward ending to the case, which ignores some complexities?
- Were my decisions consonant with and guided by wisdom, compassion, love and truth?
- How will all this influence my future practice as a clinician and a teacher?

Endnote

As Carr, D., (2002) notes, encouragingly: 'talk of spirit and the soul has proved enduring even in an age of allegedly rampant secularism'. But, of course, none of what we offer here is to suggest that such spiritual practice is simple or easy to live by. It certainly requires sustaining through an inner contemplative discipline that reaches towards understanding self, and, importantly, *seeing the heart as teaching the mind to be more sensitive, focused, energised, subtle and refined.*

We have titled this chapter: 'Mind your heart', by which we mean both that we should look after our heart, and also that we should listen to its wisdom. So, perhaps as practitioners we should at least ask ourselves in all appropriate practice situations: *Has my heart played its part?* This is emphatically only to suggest that the realm of the mind can be enriched by the wisdom of the heart (as defined in spiritual theory and practice) but *not* that it is a replacement for it.

Appendix

Appendix

Transformative Reflective Writing: An Example
The case of cholesteatoma disease.

Acknowledgement

We are grateful to Miss Sinéad Davis, consultant surgeon, whose ideas have influenced our work on how as a clinician, to craft Reflective Writing and how to explore the professional judgements and clinical thinking involved. We thank her particularly for her time and expertise in helping us create an example for this book. The clinical case we have constructed is a mixture of several patient cases. Any resemblance to a particular patient case is only by chance.

Rainbow Writing Colours

The colours now used in this process are:

BLACK   the bullet points outlining your case

The Narrative Colours
Blue 1	the **CONTEXT** of this particular case
Blue 2	the **KIND OF PERSON** you brought to the case
Green	the **PROFESSIONALISM** you brought to the case
Red	the **FORMS OF KNOWLEDGE** you brought to the case
Pink	the **THERAPEUTIC RELATIONSHIP** with the patient
Turquoise	**WIDER CONTEXTUAL AWARENESS** in the case

The Exploratory Colours
Brown	Professional Judgement
Purple	Clinical Reasoning and Deliberation

Step One: Bullet points of a consultant case. (Chapter Five)

- A 49-year-old female librarian was referred to me because of a persistent discharge from her left ear.

- Clinical examination revealed granulomatous disease in a tympanic membrane retraction pocket.

- The patient was referred for a CT scan, which confirmed the presence of cholesteatoma.

- At the clinic following the scan, I explained the findings of the scan; namely disease in the left ear (which had poor levels of hearing), but was the patient's only hearing ear.

- I discussed with one of my colleagues about proceeding with surgery on the left ear, and with another colleague about what options were available for the patient if she did go deaf in the left ear after surgery.

- I then met the patient again in outpatients' department. She was extremely anxious to go ahead with surgery as she had already spent a lot of time off work because of the condition. I agreed and the decision was made to proceed with the operation.

- During the operation on the left ear I removed the disease from the attic region of the ear but was left with the dilemma about removing the pocket over the stapes (the third hearing bone). I left the pocket undisturbed.

- At one-month post-operation the patient was recovering well from her surgery.

Step Two: Creating the Doctor-centred Narrative (Chapter Six)

A 49-year-old female librarian was referred to me because of a persistent discharge from her left ear. The history that I elicited from the patient was that she had no hearing in her right ear since birth and had recent problems with persistent discharge from her left ear.

Clinical examination revealed granulomatous disease in a tympanic membrane retraction pocket on the left side. There was no ear canal present on the right side. I sensed her anxiety and reassured her that I would do my best to relieve her problem. I explained that this would involve investigations and the possibility of an operation. I explained my suspicions to her and suggested that the next step would be to order a CT scan.

The patient was referred for a CT scan and the report indicated the presence of cholesteatoma. I reviewed the scan for myself before seeing the patient in clinic.

At the clinic following the scan, I explained to the patient the findings of the scan; namely disease in the left ear (which had poor levels of hearing), but was the patient's only hearing ear. I also explained about cholesteatomatous disease, and the possible outcome, over time, if the disease was left. I gave her the opportunity of asking any questions.

I then discussed the operation for this disease and the risks associated with the surgery (operating on the left ear could leave the patient totally deaf). The complications from surgery are very similar to the risks of leaving the disease but that by operating I hoped to minimise the risk of a complication occurring. She appeared unphased by this idea and showed some relief that something could be done. I was concerned however that she had not understood the possibility of complications.

She was anxious to go ahead with surgery, despite the risk of ending up totally deaf and appeared more concerned about getting back to work than she was about the consequences of a sudden operative complication occurring. Despite hearing complications / risks of surgery she just wanted to get on with the operation and was resigned to the fact that complications occur. Given the patient's reaction, I assumed she had not appreciated what impact a surgical complication would have, in particular the impact that total loss of hearing would have on her life. I had provided the patient with detailed information and believed that she would have been unable to process all this information immediately. I was concerned that once the patient heard about the risk of meningitis / brain abscess (which can occur, though rarely, with this condition) she had focused on this and was not giving any consideration to the other possible complications.

I also explained that one of the relative contraindications to surgery on the ear is operating on the patient's 'only hearing ear'. I explained to the patient that though I accepted her expressed desire to have surgery, that I, as her surgeon, wished to ensure that I had reviewed / considered all aspects of her complicated case before proceeding. I explained that I therefore wanted to discuss her case with my colleagues. Initially the patient seemed to be very much of the opinion that I 'knew best', but I was not so convinced. I had a limited experience as a relatively new consultant. I recognised that different surgeons would hold different opinions about whether to proceed with surgery on the left ear or not. I was concerned that my gut instinct, to operate on the patient's left ear, may not have been the opinion held by more experienced surgeons, and I wished to discuss the case with them, to reassure myself that I was doing the right thing for this patient. I had also seen the patient in the middle of a busy clinic, which had been delayed due to an earlier emergency, and was concerned that perhaps circumstances had influenced how I had imparted the information to her. Perhaps the subconscious pressure of needing to finish clinic before the afternoon consultant arrived or just a lack of clarity of thought from a time-pressured clinic had influenced how I had expressed myself on that day. I also wanted to ensure that the patient had fully considered the gravity of the situation. Before she left, I gave the patient an information leaflet about the ear disease, the surgery for this condition and its associated risks. I assumed the patient was concerned enough about her condition that she would read the information leaflet and I hoped that would clarify any issues I had not fully addressed. That way I could have a more informed discussion with the patient at her next outpatient appointment.

Though not entirey unheard of, this was the first time, as a consultant I had come across this type of case (cholesteatomatous disease in an only hearing ear). I also believed that the patient would accept 'the facts' as presented by me and would go with any decision I made. I was concerned that my initial thought (to operate on the left ear, in an attempt to preserve the patient's remaining hearing) might not have been the general consensus opinion held amongst a group of surgeons. I was anxious to do the best by my patient. I was also aware that in the event of a complication occurring and a medico-legal case arising, I wished to be certain that my decision to operate would be considered the most appropriate management for that patient. I wished to be certain that I was doing 'what was right' both for my patient and for myself (a new consultant who had a reputation to build).

I discussed with one of my colleagues about proceeding with surgery on the left ear, and with another colleague about what options were available for the patient if she did go deaf in the left ear after surgery. He first informed me he too would proceed with surgery in the left ear first, but stated that he was not sure if other ENT colleagues elsewhere would do the same. I discussed with another colleague, in another hospital, about what options for hearing rehabilitation were available for the patient if she did go deaf in the left ear after surgery. I was still concerned the patient did not have a realistic grasp of what being totally deaf would be like. I was anxious to explore, prior to proceeding with surgery, future options of providing a hearing aid (in the form of a specialist implanted hearing aid) to the patient, should the need arise. Having discussed this case with two of my colleagues, I felt confident that proceeding with surgery was the correct clinical decision in this patient's case. I also felt reassured that I had considered and explored all appropriate options when making this professional decision. I wonder how I would have felt about operating had I found out that post-operative hearing rehabilitation would not be available / appropriate for this patient.

I then met the patient again in outpatients' department. We had a detailed discussion and I felt, on this occasion, that the patient had in fact considered her options in detail. I made the decision to proceed with the operation, in keeping with the patient's wishes.

During the operation on the left ear I removed the disease from most of the middle ear cavity but was left with the dilemma about removing the pocket over the stapes (the third hearing bone). I left the pocket undisturbed. Removal of this pocket greatly increased the risk to the patient's hearing. Not removing it potentially increased the risk of recurrence of the disease. I left the pocket undisturbed. I did not wish to unduly increase the risk to the patient's hearing. My decision not to operate on that part of the ear was, in my opinion, a considered one. I based my decision partly on my sense of duty to my patient not to put her at undue risk, as there was no disease in that part of the ear at the time of surgery. I also believed that despite our discussions prior to surgery, neither the patient nor I could truly appreciate what impact it would have on her life if the patient were to be rendered totally deaf at the age of 49yrs. I thought that I would find that an extremely difficult situation and assumed finding herself totally deaf all of a sudden would have a similar impact on my patient also.

One month post-operatively, the patient is recovering well from her surgery.

Step Three: Interrogating the case narrative for Professional Judgements and Clinical thinking (Chapter Seven)

A 49-year-old female librarian was referred to me because of a persistent discharge from her left ear. The history that I elicited from the patient was that she had no hearing in her right ear since birth and had recent problems with persistent discharge from her left ear.

Clinical examination revealed granulomatous disease in a tympanic membrane retraction pocket on the left side. There was no ear canal present on the right side. I sensed her anxiety and reassured her that I would do my best to relieve her problem. I explained that this would involve investigations and the possibility of an operation. I explained my suspicions to her and suggested that the next step would be to order a CT scan. **Clinical Reasoning (1), Professional Judgement (1)**: personal professional judgement. Not all surgeons scan these patients pre-op.

The patient was referred for a CT scan and the report indicated the presence of cholesteatoma. I reviewed the scan for myself before seeing the patient in clinic.

At the clinic following the scan, I explained to the patient the findings of the scan; namely disease in the left ear (which had poor levels of hearing), but was the patient's only hearing ear. I also explained about cholesteatomatous disease, and the possible outcome, over time, if the disease was left. I gave her the opportunity of asking any questions. **Clinical Reasoning (2)**.

I then discussed the operation for this disease and the risks associated with the surgery (operating on the left ear could leave the patient totally deaf). **Clinical Reasoning (3)**. The complications from surgery are very similar to the risks of leaving the disease but by operating I hoped to minimise the risk of a complication occurring. **Clinical Reasoning (4) / Deliberation (1)**. She appeared unphased by this idea and showed some relief that something could be done. I was concerned however that she had not understood the possibility of complications.

She was anxious to go ahead with surgery, despite the risk of ending up totally deaf and appeared more concerned about getting back to work than she was about the consequences of a sudden operative complication occurring. Despite hearing complications / risks of surgery she just wanted to get on with the operation and was resigned to the fact that complications occur. Given the patient's reaction, I assumed she had not appreciated what impact a surgical complication would have, in particular the impact that a total loss of hearing would have on her life. I had provided the patient with detailed information and believed that she would have been unable to process all this information immediately. I was concerned that once the patient heard about the risk of meningitis / brain abscess (which can occur, though rarely, with this condition) she had focused on this and was not giving any consideration to the other possible complications.

I also explained that one of the relative contraindications to surgery on the ear is operating on the patient's 'only hearing ear'. **Clinical Reasoning (5)**. I explained to the patient that though I accepted her expressed desire to have surgery, that I, as her surgeon, wished to ensure that I had reviewed / considered all aspects of her complicated case before proceeding. **Deliberation (3)**. I explained that I therefore wanted to discuss her case with my colleagues. **Professional Judgement (2)**: I thought I had made a wise professional judgement here, but could it be interpreted as self-interested professional judgement? Initially the patient seemed to be very much of the opinion that I 'knew best', but I was not so convinced. I had a limited experience as a relatively new consultant. I recognised that different surgeons would hold different opinions about whether to proceed with surgery on the left ear or not. I was concerned that my gut instinct, to operate on the patient's left ear, may not have been the opinion held by more experienced surgeons, and I wished to discuss the case with them, to reassure myself that I was doing the right thing for this patient. I had also seen the patient in the middle of a busy clinic, which had been delayed due to an earlier emergency, and was concerned that perhaps circumstances had influenced how I had imparted the information to her. Perhaps the subconscious pressure of needing to finish clinic before the afternoon consultant arrived or just a lack of clarity of thought from a time-pressured clinic had influenced how I had expressed myself on that-day. I also wanted to ensure that the patient had fully considered the gravity of the situation. Before she left, I gave the patient an information leaflet about the ear disease, the surgery for this condition and its associated risks. **Deliberation (4)**. I assumed the patient was concerned enough about her condition that she would read the information leaflet and I hoped that would clarify any issues I had not fully addressed. That way I could have a more informed discussion with the patient at her next outpatient appointment. **Professional Judgement (3)**: Again was there an element of self-interest here? Or was it a wise judgement to give the patient the leaflet?

Though not entirely unheard of, this was the first time I had come across this type of case (cholesteatomatous disease in an only hearing ear) as a consultant. I also believed that the patient would accept 'the facts' as presented by me and would go with any decision I made. I was concerned that my initial thought (to operate on the left ear, in an attempt to preserve the patient's remaining hearing) might not have been the general consensus opinion held. **Deliberation (5)**. I was anxious to do the best by my patient. I was also aware that in the event of a complication occurring and a medico-legal case arising, I wished to be certain that my decision to operate would be considered the most appropriate management for that patient. I wished to be certain that I was doing 'what was right' both for my patient and for myself (a relatively junior consultant who had a reputation to build.

I discussed with one of my colleagues about proceeding with surgery on the left ear, **Deliberation (6)**. and with another colleague about what options were available for the patient if she did go deaf in the left ear after surgery. The first informed me he too would proceed with surgery in the left ear first, but stated that he was not sure if other ENT colleagues elsewhere would do the same. I discussed with another colleague, in another hospital, about what options for hearing rehabilitation were available for the patient if she did go deaf in the left ear after surgery. I was still concerned the patient did not have a realistic grasp of what being totally deaf would be like. I was anxious to explore, prior to proceeding with surgery, future options of providing a hearing aid (in the form of a specialist implanted hearing aid) to the patient, should the need arise. Having discussed this case with two of my colleagues, I felt confident that proceeding with surgery was the correct clinical decision in this patient's case. I also felt reassured that I had considered and explored all appropriate options when making this professional decision. I wonder how I would have felt about operating had I found out that post-operative hearing rehabilitation would not be available / appropriate for this patient. **Professional Judgement (4)**: Maturing / Wise judgement.

I then met the patient again in the outpatients' department. We had a detailed discussion and I felt, on this the, that the patient had in fact considered her options in detail. I made the decision to proceed with the operation, in keeping with the patient's wishes. **Professional Judgement (5)**: wise judgement.

During the operation on the left ear I removed the disease from most of the middle ear cavity but was left with the dilemma about removing the pocket over the stapes (the third hearing bone). I left the pocket undisturbed. Removal of this pocket greatly increased the risk to the patient's hearing. Not removing it potentially increased the risk of recurrence of the disease. **Deliberation (9)**. I left the pocket undisturbed. I did not wish to unduly increase the risk to the patient's hearing. My decision not to operate on that part of the ear was, in my opinion, a considered one. I based my decision partly on my sense of duty to my patient not to put her at undue risk, as there was no disease in that part of the ear at the time of surgery. I also believed that despite our discussions prior to surgery, neither the patient nor I could truly appreciate what impact it would have on her life if the patient were to be rendered totally deaf at the age of 49yrs. I thought that I would find that an extremely difficult situation and assumed finding herself totally deaf all of a sudden would have a similar impact on my patient also. **Professional Judgement (6)**: maturing judgement.

One month post-operatively, the patient is recovering well from her surgery.

Appendix

Further comments on the Professional Judgements

As the consultant of this patient I knew that this complex case required me to make many professional judgements along the way. My first judgement of this case was where I made a decision to refer my patient for a CT scan prior to deciding on the appropriate management of her condition. (**Professional Judgement 1**) Not every consultant requests CT scans pre-op but my decision to do so was based on the belief that a scan could offer more information regarding the nature/extent of the disease. Given the complexity of this patient's case, I wanted to be sure I knew the full extent of her disease to be able to share this with her and allow it to inform my intended action and thus I felt doing the test was in her best interests.

When I next met with the patient, it was clear she wished to proceed with surgery without further delay. She wanted to get back to work as soon as possible. However, I decided not to agree to her request immediately. I decided to defer my decision on management until I had discussed her case with my colleagues (**Professional Judgement 2**). In this instance it is possible to believe that I was in fact acting out of self-interest, as my choice of decision was designed to enhance my own performance and achievement. I did not want to make the wrong decision. At the time of making my judgement I believed it was because I was aware of the 'lottery' effect and did not want the patient to 'suffer' due to my decision. However, it is clear I also had the worry of medico-legal issues in mind. I was concerned not just that I was making the right decision for this patient, but that I would be seen to have done so by my peers and would be able to defend my decision (to operate on this woman's left ear) to my opponents (those who would not proceed with surgery in this case) if called to do so. My decision in part therefore must be considered to be a self-defensive judgement.

Having made my decision to discuss this patient's case with my colleagues, I proceeded to give my patient an information leaflet on the disease and surgery (**Professional Judgement 3**). This is not something I do for all my patients (as I often fear the information will scare them too much) but on this occasion I deliberately decided to give the patient the information. Again, on reflection, I can question whether this was based on wise judgement (believing that providing this patient with all available information was in her best interests). Perhaps instead it was a self-defensive judgement, allowing me to work through my clinic as efficiently as possible (rather than taking even more time to talk to my patient); while still making me feel like I have done something for my patient?

My decision to discuss with a colleague the options available for hearing rehabilitation (**Professional Judgement 4**) though were done with the patient's best interests at heart (Wise Judgement) and showing perhaps signs of maturing judgement and enlightenment, but it did at the same time, I think, put me at risk of scorn from some colleagues by exposing what might have been seen as a weakness on my part. I believe that I was wise in considering the future options available to my patient but at the time was questioning myself about my reason for doing this. Was I pursuing this in order to reassure myself about what else that could still be done for her, in the event of a complication arising? By exploring this before surgery, I offering my colleague the opportunity to undertake the primary surgery if he felt that was the right thing to do. It therefore appeared that I was considering my patient's interests above all else but, in reality, did I approach this colleague because I needed to be sure, for me, that I was doing all that I could. My decision was therefore not entirely wise maybe even a self-defensive one.

Finally, I did decide to operate on this patient, having satisfied my own and the patient's questions about this case (**Professional Judgement 5**): Wise Judgement. But, as is so often the case, just when it seems an answer has been found another unexpected situation arises. On this occasion, having no further opportunity to engage in collaborative conversation with my patient, I was faced with an unexpected finding during the operation. Intraoperative decision making is part of the role of the surgeon. At the time I felt like my management decision, once again, held the potential for disaster either way. My patient could, if I proceeded to try to remove this pocket of disease entirely, be left deaf immediately after the surgery or she could be left with an area (the pocket) in which disease could reoccur, potentially causing a complication at a later date. I decided to leave the pocket intact to be observed in clinic in the years to come (**Professional Judgement 6**). Once again at the time of surgery I believed that I had made a wise judgement, with the patient's best interests at heart. There was no disease in that area at that time, and operating could have had drastic consequences (leaving the patient totally deaf). Perhaps, on reflection, my decision may have been a little more about playing it safe for me (maturing judgement) than I would at first have admitted?

Further comments on the Clinical Thinking

In my management of this patient, I firstly framed the case by gathering information about the patient's history and by recording my clinical examination findings. Having completed my initial assessment I immediately began my clinical reasoning stating '... my suspicions' and taking the decision to investigate further by referring the patient for a CT scan (**Clinical Reasoning 1**).

I continued my clinical reasoning during that initial consultation by explaining to the patient about this type of ear disease, its natural progression and associated risks, as well as informing her about the management options and surgery. These points were all raised in discussion of the disease and surgery in general (**Clinical Reasoning 2, 3 and 4**) but I immediately found myself considering the impact of the present on this patient who only had one functioning ear (in terms of hearing). I hoped to minimise the risk to the patient by performing surgery but it is clear from my use of language both to the patient and here in my discussion that I was not convinced that that would in fact be the outcome (**Deliberation 1**).

Again I reverted to clinical reasoning and discussion with the patient; discussing the golden rule of ear surgery (never operate on the patient's ear, if it is the only ear they can hear with) (**Clinical Reasoning 5**). I believe my main reason for doing so was firstly so that the patient could have all the facts in order to make her decision regarding her management. I also believe that by having these discussions I was hoping to glean further information about the patient; her values, wishes and perhaps also determine her ability to make a fully informed decision (**Deliberation 2**). I was at this point putting myself at risk of being seen by the patient as perhaps 'unsure' of what I should do. I weighed up that it was better to be in full knowledge of the facts and share with her all the potential risks.

This lead me on to my own deliberation 'as her surgeon' of this 'complicated case' (**Deliberation 3**). Did I have enough experience on which to base my decision regarding this patient's management? What would my colleagues do if faced with the same case? I was anxious that the patient's management was not influenced by the lottery of her seeing me rather than another of my consultant colleagues in outpatient clinic.

I recognised that I can express myself better on some occasions that on others. I pondered the fact that my ability to express myself when under time-pressure in a delayed clinic might have influenced the patient's decision unduly. Had my explanation been clear enough on this occasion so as to allow me to obtain fully informed consent at that time? My deliberation on these issues (**Deliberation 4**) caused me to offer the patient written information regarding her condition, such that she could review this information later. Thus I hoped that when I next met the patient I would be able to have a more detailed and informed collaborative discussion with her.

I deliberated on the medico-legal aspects of the case. If a complication did arise, would I be able to defend my decision to the patient, to myself or in a court of law? Had I taken every possible step to ensure I was offering the best possible care to this patient? (**Deliberation 5**)

In order to ensure that I could defend my decision, I chose to involve other professional colleagues in my deliberation. With one of my colleagues, I discussed whether the patient should have surgery on this left ear at all (**Deliberation 6**). I subsequently discussed with another colleague, based at a different hospital, if the option of rehabilitation would be available to this patient if a complication arose during surgery. I believed that knowing whether an option for hearing rehabilitation was available to my patient could influence her / my decision to proceed (**Deliberation 7**). I also understood that it is often easier to do a second operation on a patient's ear if you have performed the primary surgery. Knowing I could not perform the implant surgery required for rehabilitation, I therefore discussed the option of the implant surgeon performing the primary surgery also (**Deliberation 8**). He felt this was not necessary in this patient's case. I found this supportive and reassuring.

Armed with this information I met with the patient again. Once again we entered the clinical reasoning phase; discussing her understanding of the disease and her wishes regarding her condition (**Clinical Reasoning 6**). With a greater understanding of my patient and her wishes, as well as a greater confidence in my own understanding of the case, I then deliberated further (**Deliberation 9**) and was able to arrive at a (product) professional judgement during that meeting in outpatients.

My decision making did not end there however. During the surgery I was once again faced with a number of unexpected issues. The extent of the disease and the area of the ear involved forced me to consider the option of not operating on / removing all the disease (**Clinical Reasoning 7**). On this occasion I considered the possible outcomes regarding removal / leaving the disease, in light of my knowledge of the patient and her wishes. I weighed this up in the light of my own experience and understanding of how this 'pocket' disease differed from the expected disease (cholesteatoma) (**Deliberation 10**). I made a professional decision to leave this less aggressive disease in situ and to monitor it in the future, thus minimising the risks to this patient at this time.

Step Four: Summary (Chapter Eight)

I have summarized my key learning points below as a series of bullet points. They are in no particular order of priority but I believe each offers a specific point.

- When I first started Reflective Writing I found it quite time-consuming. However, as I have become more familiar with the process it not only influences how I write but how I think in clinical practice.
- The writing has helped me clarify my thinking and therefore be more confident and articulate in explaining to others my argument for my actions.
- In this case I was surprised how many times I seemed to be exercising with the patient my thoughts on clinical reasoning. It caused me to consider how time-pressures might influence my patience in doing this. My deliberation prior to the surgery about this case helped considerably my need for an 'on the hoof' deliberative decision during the actual operation. This is something I must remember to highlight when teaching young surgeons.
- I was surprised at how many judgements I made and this has sharpened my listening to trainees (and others!) about how they relate their actions and decision making. It has changed how I ask them questions. I now want to them first to explain 'what they think they should do in a particular patient case' (Final step of the Clinical Thinking Pathway), rather than starting at the top end of the Clinical Thinking Pathway (the standard way of offering a case). I now expect my trainees to start their response to me on ward rounds and in clinic when presenting a case, at the end of the clinical thinking pathway, leaving me to tease out of them the clinical reasoning and deliberation they engaged with along that pathway. At first they do not find this easy because it is not what they are used to!
- This piece is a useful teaching resource.
- I believe this piece would be useful as evidence for my appraisal for demonstrating my commitment to: Communications, Partnership and Teamwork and Maintaining Trust.
- I now have experience that this can be educational when as a team activity each member shares their own Rainbow Writing for discussion.

References

References

Alexander, R. (2004) *Towards Dialogic Teaching*. Cambridge: Dialogos.

Barnes, D. (1995) The Role of Talk in Learning, in K. Norman (ed) Thinking Voices: *The work of the National Oracy Project*. London: Hodder & Stoughton.

Bauman, Z. (2000) *Liquid Modernity*. Cambridge: Polity.

Bawa-Garba   https://www.bmj.com/bawa-garba.

Benner, P. (1984) *From Novice to Expert: Excellence and power in Clinical Nursing Practice*. London: Addison Wesley Publishing Company.

Biesta, G. (2010) *Good Education in an Age of Measurement: Ethics, Politics, Democracy*. London: Routledge.

Blond, P., Antonacopoulou, E. and Pabst, A. (2015) *In Professions We Trust: Fostering Virtuous Practitioners in Teaching, Law and Medicine*. London: ResPublica. Available via: http://www.respublica.org.uk/wp-content/uploads/2015/02/In-Professions-We-Trust.pdf

Bolton, G. (2014) *Reflective Practice Writing and Professional Development*. London: Sage Publications.

Bolton, G., Delderfield, R. (2018) *Reflective Practice: Writing and Professional Development*. London: Sage Publications. Fourth Edition.

Boniface, G., Fish, D. (2012). Reconfiguring professional thinking and conduct: A challenge for occupational therapists in practice. G. Boniface, A. Seymour. (eds) *Using Occupational Therapy Theory in Practice*. Blackwell Publishing Ltd.

Boniface, G., Seymour, A. (2012) *Using Occupational Therapy Theory in Practice*. Blackwell Publishing Ltd.

Boud, D., Keogh, R. and Walker, D. (1985) *Reflection: Turning Experience into Learning*. London: Sage Publications.

Bourgeault, C. (2003) *The Wisdom Way of Knowing: Reclaiming an Ancient Tradition to awaken the heart*. San Francisco: Jossey Bass.

Bourgeault, C. (2016) *The Heart of Centering Prayer: non-dual Christianity in theory and practice*. Boulder, Colorado: Shambhala Publications.

Broadfoot, P. (1996) Educational Assessment: The myth of measurement, in P. Woods (ed) *Contemporary Issues in teaching and learning*. London: RoutledgeFalmer.

Brown, J., Leadbetter, P., & Clabburn, O. (2016). *An evaluation at East Lancashire Hospitals Trust (ELHT) of the impact of the project: Supervision Matters: Clinical Supervision for Quality Medical Care*. Health Education England (North West).

Bullock, A., Hardyman, J. and Phillips, S. (2012) *Quality Teaching and Learning in clinical practice for F2 Teachers and Learners*: Cardiff: Cardiff University.

Campbell, A. (1984) *Moderated Love: A Theology of Professional Care*. London: SPCK.

Carper, Barbara. (1978) Fundamental Patterns of Knowing in Nursing. *Advances in Nursing Science*: Vol 1; Issue 1: 13-24.

Carr, D. (2002) Moral education and the perils of developmentalism. *Journal of Moral Education*. Vol. 30, pp. 5-19.

Carr, D. (2003) Rival conceptions of practice in education and teaching. *Journal of Philosophy of Education*. Vol. 37, No 2, pp. 253-266.

Carr, W., Kemmis, S. (1986) *Becoming Critical: Education, Knowledge and Action Research*. London, Falmer.

Carr, W. (1995) What is an Educational Practice? *For Education: Towards Critical Educational Enquiry*. Buckingham: Open University Press.

Charon, R. (2006) *Narrative Medicine: Honoring the Stories of Illness*. Oxford: Oxford University Press.

Clandinin, D.J., Connelly, F.M. (2000) *Narrative Inquiry: Experience and story in Qualitative Research*. San Francisco: Jossey Bass.

Cobb, M., Dowrick, C., Lloyd-Williams, Mari. (2012) What Can We Learn About the Spiritual Needs of Palliative Care Patients From the Research Literature? *Journal of Pain and Symptom Management*. Vol; 43: 1105-1119.

de Cossart, L., Fish D. (2002) Membership of a profession. Part Two: The nature of professional knowledge in medical practice. *Mersey Deanery Newsletter* vol: 14 No 2. Liverpool: Mersey Deanery.

de Cossart, L., and Fish, D. (2005) *Cultivating a Thinking Surgeon: new perspectives on clinical teaching, learning and assessment*. Shrewsbury: TfN Press.

de Cossart, L., Fish D. (2006a) Thinking outside the (tick) box: Rescuing professionalism and professional judgement. *Medical Education* Vol: 40: 403–4.

de Cossart, L., Fish, D. (2006b) So just how do surgeons think? *Hospital Doctor*, 27th April, pp: 20-21.

de Cossart, L., Fish, D. (eds) (2011) *Enhancing Teaching and Learning in Postgraduate Medicine.* The proceedings of the Jephcott symposium on the Invisibles at the Royal Society of Medicine in April 2010. London: Royal Society of Medicine.

de Cossart, L., Fish D., Hillman K. (2012) Clinical Reflection: a vital process for supporting the development of wisdom in doctors. *Current Opinion in Critical Care.* Vol 18 No 6 :712-7.

de Cossart, L and Fish, D. (2013) Worthwhile Education: a vision for Educational Leadership. In *Excellence in Medical Education* (AoME): Issue 4.

de Cossart, L. Fish, D., Thomé, R. (2013) Education for Clinical Teachers: Does it make a difference? In *Excellence in Medical Education* (AoME): Issue 1.

Cox, K. (1999) *Doctor and Patient: exploring clinical thinking.* Sydney: University of New South Wales Press.

Dawes, J. (2017) *Discernment and Inner knowing: making decisions for the best.* FeedARead.com Publishing.

Dewey, J. (1897) My pedagogic creed. *The School Journal.* LIV (3): Jan 16: 77-80 (http://www.infed.org/archives/e-texts/e-dew-pc.htm).

Dewey, J. (1910) *How We Think.* New York: Dover Publications Inc. (Revised 1933)

Dewey, J. (1916) *Democracy and Education.* New York: Free Press.

Department of Health, *Modernising Medical Careers.* (February 2003), The Statutory Office: London. (www.doh.gov.uk).

Downie, R.S., Macnaughton, J. (2001) *Clinical Judgement: Evidence in practice.* Oxford: Oxford University Press.

Driscoll, J. (2000) *Practising Clinical Supervision: a reflective approach.* Edinburgh: Ballière.

Easwaran, E., (2007) *The Bhagavad Gita.* Califormia: Nilgiri Press. (Second Edition).

Eliot, TS. (2001) *Four Quartets.* London: Faber and Faber.

Epstein, R.M. (1999) Mindful Practice. *The Journal of the American Medical Association.* V.ol:

282; No 9: 833-839.

Eraut, M. (1995) Schön Shock: a case for re-framing reflection in action? *Teachers and Training: Theory and Practice*. Vol: 1 No1: 9-23.

Fish, D. (1998) *Appreciating Practice in the Caring Professions: Refocusing Professional Development and Practitioner Research*. Oxford: Butterworth Heinemann.

Fish, D. (2005) The Anatomy of Evaluation. In M. Rose, and D. Best (eds.) *Understanding Supervision in Health Science Education and Practice*. Edinburgh: Elsevier.

Fish. D. (2009) Research as a pragmatic practice in B. Green, (ed) *Understanding and Researching Professional Practice*. Rotterdam: Sense Publications.

Fish, D. (2012a) *Refocusing Postgraduate Medical Education: from the technical to the moral mode of practice*. Cranham: Aneumi Publications.

Fish, D. (2012b) From Strands to The Invisibles, in Boniface, G & Seymour, A. (eds)) *Using Occupational Therapy Theory in Practice*. Oxford: Blackwell Publishing Ltd.

Fish, D. (2015) *Starting with myself as doctor and a supervisor*. Booklet 1 of Medical Supervision Matters, Aneumi Publications, Cranham, UK.

Fish, D., Brigley, S. (2010) Exploring the Practice of Education. In J. Higgs, D. Fish, I. Goulter, S. Loftus, J-A. Reid and F. Trede (eds), *Education for Future Practice*. Rotterdam: Sense Publications, p:113-122.

Fish, D., Coles, C. (eds) (1998) *Developing Professional Judgement in Health Care: Learning Through the Critical Appreciation of Practice*. Oxford: Butterworth-Heinemann.

Fish, D., Coles, C. (2005) *Medical Education: Developing a curriculum for practice*. Maidenhead: Open University Press.

Fish, D., de Cossart, L. (2007) *Developing the Wise Doctor*. London: Royal Society of Medicine Press.

Fish, D. de Cossart, L (2013) *Reflection for Medical Appraisal*. Cranham: Aneumi Publications.

Fish, D. de Cossart, L. (2019) Cultivating a Thinking Surgeon, using a Clinical Thinking Pathway as a Learning and Assessment Process: Ten years on. In eds J Higgs, G Jensen, S Loftus, N Christensen. *Clinical Reasoning in the Health Professions*. Edinburgh: Elsevier. (Fourth Edition)

Fish, D. de Cossart, L., and Wright, T. (2015a) *Practical dilemmas about supervision and teaching*. Booklet 2 of Medical Supervision Matters. Aneumi Publications, Cranham, UK.

Fish, D. de Cossart, L., and Wright, T. (2015b) *Practical Dilemmas about the learner and learning*. Booklet 3 of Medical Supervision Matters. Aneumi Publications, Cranham, UK.

Fish, D. de Cossart, L., and Wright, T. (2015c) *Practical Dilemmas about Assessment and Evaluation*. Booklet 4 of Medical Supervision Matters. Aneumi Publications, Cranham, UK.

Fish, D., Higgs, J. (2007) The context of clinical decision-making in the Twenty First Century. In: J. Higgs, M. Jones, S. Loftus, N. Christensen. eds. *Clinical Reasoning in the Health Professions*. Edinburgh: Elsevier. (Third Edition).

Fish, D., Twinn, S. (1997) *Quality Clinical Supervision in the Health Care Profession*. Oxford: Butterworth Heinemann.

Fish, D. Twinn, S., Purr, B. (1990) *How to enable learning through professional practice: a cross-profession investigation of the supervision of preservice practice. Report Number Two*. London: West London Institute: College of Brunel University.

Frank, A. (1995) *The Wounded Story Teller: Body, Illness and Ethics*. Chicago and London: University of Chicago Press.

Freeth, D., Hammick, M., Koppel, I., Reeves, S., & Barr, H. (2005). *Effective Interprofessional Education*. Oxford: Blackwell Publishing.

Freidson, E. (1994) *Professionalism Reborn: Theory, Prophecy and Policy*. Oxford: Polity Press.

Freidson, E. (2001) *Professionalism: The Third Way*. Oxford: Polity Press.

Freire, P. (1970) *Pedagogy of the oppressed*. Harmondsworth, United Kingdom: Penguin Books.

Freire, P. (1998) 'Challenging the banking concept of education' in *Pedagogy of the Oppressed*. New York: Continuum Books.

Gawande, A. (2001) *Complications: A surgeon's notes on an Imperfect Science*. London: Profile Books.

General Medical Council (GMC, 2013). *Good Medical Practice*. www.gmc-uk.org/guidance.

General Medical Council (GMC, 2018) *Reflective Practice*. https://www.gmc-uk.org/education/standards-guidance-and-curricula/guidance/the-reflective-practitioner-guidance-for-doctors-and-medical-students

General Medical Council (GMC, 2019) *Generic Professional Capabilities Framework.* https://www.gmc-uk.org/-/media/documents/generic-professional-capabilities-framework-0817_pdf-70417127.pdf

Gibbs, G. (1988) *Learning by Doing. A Guide to Teaching and Learning Methods.* Further Education Unit, Oxford Polytechnic, Oxford.

Greenhalgh, T., Hurwitz, B,. (1998) (eds.) *Narrative Based Medicine: Dialogue and Discourse in Clinical Practice.* London: BMJ Books.

Greenwood, J. (1993) Reflective Practice: a critique of the work of Argyris and Schön, *Journal of Advanced Nursing.* Vol 18: 1183-1187

Griffiths Report (https://www.bmj.com/content/bmj/287/6402/1391.full.pdf

Grundy, S. (1987) *The Curriculum: Product or Praxis.* London, Falmer Press.

Habermas, J. (1971) *Towards a Rational Society.* Trans. J.J. Shappiro, London: Heinemann.

Habermas, J. (1972) *Knowledge and Human Interest.* Trans. J.J. Shappiro, London: Heinemann.

Habermas J. (1974) *Theory and Practice.* Trans, J. Viertel, London: Heinemann.

Hansen, D. (2001) *Exploring the Moral Heart of Teaching: Towards a Teacher's Creed.* New York: Teachers College Press.

Higgs, J. (1990) Fostering the Acquisition of Clinical reasoning skills. *New Zealand Journal of Occupational Therapy,* December 1990, pp 13-18.

Higgs, J. (2003) 'Do you reason like a (health) professional? In G. Brown, S. Esdaile, S. Ryan. (eds) *Becoming an Advanced Practitioner*, Edinburgh, Butterworth Heinemann. (chapter 6 pp. 144 – 160.)

Higgs, J., Fish, D. and Rothwell, R. (2004) 'Practice knowledge — critical appreciation'. In J. Higgs, B. Richardson, M. Abrandt Dahlgren. (eds) *Developing Practice Knowledge for Health Professionals*, Edinburgh, Butterworth Heinemann.

Higgs, J. and Jones, M. (Eds) (2002) *Clinical Reasoning in the Health Professions.* (Second Edition). Oxford, Butterworth Heinemann.

Hordern, J. (2018) Covenant, compassion and marketisation in healthcare: the mastery of mammon and the service of grace. In T. Feiler, J. Hordern, A. Papanikitas, A. (eds) *Marketisation, Ethics and Healthcare.* London: Routledge. (Chapter 7)

References

Horujy, S.S. Stoeckl, Kristina, Jakim, Boris. (2015) *Practices of the Self and Spiritual Practices: Michel Foucault and the Eastern Christian Discourse.* Michigan, USA, Wm. B. Eerdmans Publishing Company.

HRH Prince Charles. (2006) *The Sacred Web: A Journal of Tradition and Modernity*: Sept 23rd - 24th). http://www.sacredweb.com/conference06/conference_introduction.html

Hoyle, E. (1974) Professionality, professionalism and the control of teaching, *London Educational Review.* Vol: 3 ; No 2: 3-18.

Hunter, K. (1993) *Doctors Stories: The Narrative Structure of Medicine.* Princeton: Princeton University Press.

Huxley, A. (1945) *The Perennial Tradition.* USA, Harper and Brothers.

Iliffe, S. (2008) *From General Practice to Primary Care: The Industrialisation of Family Medicine.* Oxford: Oxford University Press.

Irvine, Donald. (2003) *The Doctors' Tale: Professionalism and Public Trust.* Radcliffe Medical Press.

Irvine, D. (2018) *Medical Professionalism and the Public Interest: Reflections on a Life in Medicine.* London: Royal College of General Practitioners Heritage Committee.

Jasper, M., Rosser, M., Mooney, G. (2013). *Professional Development, Reflection and Decision-Making in Nursing and Healthcare (Advanced Healthcare Practice).* Chichester, John Wiley and Sons Ltd.

Johns, C. (1995) Framing learning through reflection within Carper's fundamental ways of knowing in nursing. *Journal of Advanced Nursing.* Vol: 22; No 2: 226–34.

Keating, T. (2001) *Journey to the Center: A Lenten Passage.* Chicago: Independent Publishers Group.

Kolb, D. (1984) *Experiential Learning as the science of learning and development.* Englewood Cliffs, New Jersey, Prentice Hall.

Launer, J. (2015) What's the point of reflective writing? *Postgraduate Medical Journal.* Vol: 91: P 1076.

Launer, J. (2019) Osler Centenary Papers: Equanimity 2020. *Postgraduate Medical Journal.* Vol: 95: P 1130.

MacIntyre, A. (1981) *After Virtue.* Paris: University of Notre Dame Press. (Third edition).

Mahendran, A. O. (2020) *Moments of Rupture: The Importance of Affect in Medical Education and Surgical Training*. London: Routledge, 'in press'.

Mann, K. (2006) Learning and Teaching in Professional Character Development, in N. Kenny and W. Shelton (eds) *Lost Virtue: Professional Character Development in Medical Education* (Advances in Bioethics Volume 10). Amsterdam: Elsevier JAI Press.

Marcotte, L., Moriates, C., Wolfson, D., Frankel, R. (2020) Professionalism as the Bedrock of High-Value Care. *Academic Medicine*. Vol 95: (6): P 864-867.

Mercer, N. (1995/2008) *The Guided Construction of Knowledge: talk amongst teachers and learners*. Bristol: Multilingual Matters Ltd.

Mercer, N. (2000) *Words and Minds: How we use language to think together*. London: Routledge.

Mercer, N. & Hodgkinson, S. (2008) (eds) *Exploring Talk in School: inspired by the work of Douglas Barnes*. London: Sage.

Douglas, M. (1987) *How Institutions Think*. Syracuse: Syracuse University Press.

Mattingly, C., Fleming M. (1994). *Clinical Reasoning: Forms of Inquiry in a Therapeutic Practice*. Philadelphia, PA: F.A. Davis Press.

Montgomery, K. (2006) *How Doctors Think: Clinical Judgement and the Practice of Medicine*. Oxford: Oxford University Press.

Moon, J. (1999) *Reflection in Learning and Professional development: Theory and Practice*. London: Kogan Page.

Murphy, N. (2002) Integrated Learning and Assessment – The Role of Learning Theories. In P. Woods, (ed) (1996) *Contemporary issues in teaching and Learning*. London: Routledge in association with the Open University.

O'Neill, O. (2002) *A Question of Trust*. Cambridge: Cambridge University Press. (The 2002 Reith Lectures).

Oakeshott, M. (1959) *On Human Conduct*. Oxford: Clarendon Books.

Oakley, M (2019) *My Sour-sweet Days*. London: SPCK Publishing.

Palmer, Parker, J. (1998) *The Courage to Teach*. San Francisco: Jossey Bass.

Pereira Grey, D. (2002) Deprofessionalising doctors? *BMJ* Vol: 324: P 627–8.

Picasso. Pablo Picasso. Paintings, Quotes and Biography. https://www.pablopicasso.org (accessed 02/06/2020).

Pollock, A.M. (2004) *NHS plc: the Privatisation of our Health Care*. London: Verso.

Pring, R. (2000) *Philosophy of Educational Research*. London: Continuum Books.

Proctor, B. (1986) Supervision: a cooperative exercise in accountability. In M. Marken, and M. Paynes, (eds.) *Enabling and Ensuring - supervision in practice*. Leicester: National Youth Bureau, Council for Education and Training in Youth and Community Work.

Rolfe, G., Jasper, Melanie., Freshwater, Dawn. (2001) *Critical Reflection for Nursing and the Helping Professions*. London, Red Globe Press.

Royal College of Physicians (RCP) (2005) *Doctors in Society, Medical Professionalism in a Changing World: Report of a Working Party*. London: Royal College of Physicians.

Ryan, S. (1995) Teaching Reasoning to Occupational Therapists during Fieldwork Education. In J. Higgs, and M. Jones (eds.) *Clinical Reasoning in the Health Professions*. (First Edition). Oxford: Butterworth Heinemann.

Schön, D. (1983) *The Reflective Practitioner*. New York: Basic Books.

Schön, D. (1987a) *Educating the Reflective Practitioner*. New York: Jossey Bass.

Schön, D. (1987b) Changing Patterns of Inquiry in Work and Living. *Journal of the Royal Society of Arts*. Vol: 135 (5367) pp: 225-237.

Schön, D. (ed.) (1991) *The Reflective Turn: case studies in and on educational practice*. New York: The Teachers College Press.

Schwartz, B. Sharpe, K. (2011) *Practical Wisdom: The Right Way to Do the Right Thing*. New York. Riverhead Books.

Seddon, J. (2008) *Systems Thinking in the Public Sector*. London: Triarchy Press.

Seldon, A. (2009) *Trust: How We Lost It And How To Get It Back*. London: Backbite Publishing.

Sokol, D. (2007). Can deceiving patients be morally acceptable? *BMJ*. Vol: 334 (7601): p 984–986.

Southern, G. Braithwaite, J. (1998) The End of Professionalism? in Social Science and Medicine. Vol: 46; No 1: p 23-28. (Also, abridged in: C. Davies, L. Findlay and A. Bullman (eds.) (2000) *Changing Practice in Health and Social Care*. London: Open University in association with Sage Publications: 300-307.)

Stenhouse, L. (1975) *An Introduction to Curriculum Research and Development.* London: Heinemann.

The Academy of Medical Royal Colleges/COPMeD publication *Reflective practice toolkit* (2018).
(www.aomrc.org.uk/wp.../Reflective_Practice_Toolkit_AoMRC_CoPMED_0818.pdf)

Thomé, R. (2012) *Educational Practice Development: An evaluation (An exploration of the impact on participants and their shared organistion of a Postgraduate Certificate in Education for Postgraduate Medical Practice 2010-2011).* Cranham: Aneumi Publications.

Thomé, R. (2013) *Educational Practice Development: An Evaluation: An exploration of the impact on participants and their shared organisation of year two of the Postgraduate Masters in Education for Postgraduate Medical Practice.* Cranham: Aneumi Publications.

Urban, D.V. (2018) Ignation Inscape and Instress in Gerard Manly Hopkin's Pied Beauty, *God's Grandeur, The Star Light Night and The Windhover:* Hopkins movement towards Igantius by way of Walter Pater. Religions, Vol: 9: p 49.

Van Manen, M. (1977) Linking ways of knowing with ways of being. *Curriculum Inquiry.* Vol: 6; p 205-88.

Van Manen, M. (1991) *The Tact of Teaching.* New York: The State of New York Press.

Van Manen, M. (2015) *Pedagogical Tact.* London: Routledge.

Wattis, J., Curran, Stephen., Rogers, M. (2017) *Spiritually Competent Practice in Healthcare.* London, UK, CRC Press Taylor and Francis Group.

Wattis, John, Rogers, Melanie, Ali, Gulnar and Curran, Stephen (2019) Bringing Spirituality and Wisdom into Practice. In: *Practice Wisdom: Values and Interpretations.* Practice Futures, Vol 3 p. 155-170. Brill, Leiden, the Netherlands.

Welby, J. (2016) *Dethroning Mammon: making money serve grace.* London: Bloomsbury Continuum.

Welby, J. (2018) *Reimagining Britain.* London: Bloomsbury Continuum.

Wells, G. (2009), *The Meaning Makers: Learning to Talk and Talking to Learn.* Bristol: Multilingual Matters, 2nd Edition.

West, L. (2001) *Doctors on the Edge: General Practitioners, Health and Learning in the Inner City.* London: Free Association Books.

White, S. and Stancombe, J. (2003). *Clinical Judgement in the Health and Welfare*

Professions: extending the evidence base. Maidenhead: Open University Press.

Wilkinson, R., Pickett, K. (2010) *The Spirit Level.* Harmondsworth, London, Penguin.

Wright, T., Fish, D. (2015) *Practical Dilemmas about Assessment and Evaluation.* Booklet 4 of Medical Supervision Matters. Aneumi Publications, Cranham, UK.

Yule, S., Flin, R., Paterson-Brown, S., Maran, N. (2006) Non-technical skills in the operating room: a review of the literature. *Surgery* Vol: 139 No: 2; p 140- 9.

Index

Academy of Medical Royal Colleges (AoMRC) 1
aims and intentions ix, 154, 175, 176
appraisal 64, 72, 117, 170-171
    GMC domains 118
Aristotle/Aristotelian 18-19, 168-181
    See also wisdom of the heart 164, 175-177, 180-182, 191-192
assessment 27, 29, 34, 50, 125-126, 136-139
audience 50, 92-93, 156
authenticity 93, 99-100
authority 17, 37, 83, 168, 186-188

Bawa Gaba 14
Being, Knowing, Doing, Thinking and Becoming 177
Bullet points 52, 54, 69-73

capabilities/capability 1, 25, 70, 75, 127, 149
capacity i, xv, 21, 53, 70, 119, 166-168, 173, 188
Care Quality Commission (CQC) 18
Chaplaincy Ward Visitors 190
character 4, 11, 18, 36, 62, 129, 133, 137-138, 165, 183
character and virtue 18
characteristics of reflective practice 33
clinical decision making 52-53, 56, 63, 99-107
Clinical Reasoning 4, 9, 99-115, 118, 179, 185, 207
Clinical Thinking Pathway 56, 63, 100-103, 207
Cloud of Unknowing 180
commitment to professionalism 3, 71
competence 30, 82, 104
components inter relate 49, 53
conduct 9, 11-12, 14, 17, 19, 24-26, 28, 46, 52, 80, 123, 126, 136, 177, 179, 183
Conversations of mankind 23
COPMeD 142
criticality 31, 36
critique 2, 11, 19-20, 24, 33, 38, 49-50, 91, 118, 124, 131
curriculum 26, 29, 43, 125, 129-131, 143-144, 148, 150-151

debate 42, 178
deep learning 50, 167
deliberation 56, 60, 63-64, 104, 123, 143, 178-179
deliberative 12, 31, 104-105, 120, 207
dialogic 32, 52, 129, 148, 152, 154-155, 160
Dialogue 32, 42, 104, 132, 134-135, 154, 180
discernment 21, 168, 180-182
Discernment and inner knowing 177
Discernment of the heart 177, 180
Discretionary 31, 104
Dis-ease in the medical profession 9, 11, 14, 16-17, 170
    The first four viewpoints 12
    A fifth view point 14
Doctor centred 54, 67, 75, 197

Educational philosophy 9, 23, 130, 146
Educational values 131
Educationally transformative 44, 46
Educationally worthwhile 70, 133, 141, 143, 145
Eliot TS 107, 167
emancipatory 70
ethical 14, 24, 33, 41, 84, 157, 184
eudemonia (human flourishing) 19
extended/restricted professional 82
evidence of progress 105, 151
    crystallising reflective evidence 171

Final Summary 52
Focus for reflection 28
Formulaic 16, 63, 104-105
General Medical Council (GMC) 75, 171
Generating knowledge out of practice 29
Generic Professional Capabilities 70, 75
good practice 24, 29, 126, 146
good teaching 125, 138
    heart of 135
Heuristic 4, 58-61
    new heuristic 191
Historical perspectives (of reflection) 37
human flourishing (see eudemonia) 19
human interests 40
human nourishment 23
Huxley 178, 180

Iceberg of practice 61
imperturbability 21, 166, 170
implications of practice 31
informal assessment 138, 158
inscape 176
insights 5, 21, 53, 56-57, 67, 71, 99-100, 115, 117, 119, 136-137, 148, 151, 172, 178, 185
integrity 25, 127
intellectually attentive 25, 127
intelligent reflection 9
Intuition 80-81, 118, 177
Introductory programme for TRP 141, 144

key thinkers 37-39, 42
Knowledge
    forms of 40, 59, 62, 64, 87, 172
Knowledge cards 59, 86

Learners' being and becoming 26
Learning conversation 130, 133-134
liberate thinking 24
Liquid modernity 183
long-term aim 1, 3, 5, 163

Maintaining trust 119-120, 171-172, 207
Malaise 13
managers 55, 57, 92, 120, 169
maturing judgement 106, 110, 112, 202-204
Medical Reflective Writing 2, 6, 63
Mind your heart 175, 192
mindfulness 41, 182
mode of practice 15, 23, 25-26, 123, 128-129, 132-133, 135, 137-138, 146
Modernising Medical Careers 15
Monet 61, 78
moral agency 2-3, 20-21, 54-55, 71, 130, 163, 165
moral mode of educational practice 125-126, 132, 163
morale 4
morally attentive to learners 25, 127
motivation 3-4, 9, 21, 24, 39, 43, 106-107, 136, 141, 163, 165

narrative (definition) 41
narrative reflection 20
nature of educational practice 25
nature of medical practice 2, 34, 164
nature of professional practice 42
New insights 56, 67, 71, 148-149, 151
Nicomachean Ethics 178
nuances 1, 9, 27, 41, 52, 63, 132, 142, 152
nurture 24, 26, 67, 89, 167, 173, 176
nurture the learner using assessment 125, 136

other professionals 1, 2, 191
Osler 166, 170
Our broken society 183
our educational philosophy 9, 23

patient care 14, 16, 34-35, 67, 103, 131, 168
Perennial Philosophy 180, 187
Perennial Tradition 178, 180, 189

Index

Personal Professional Judgement 102, 103, 108
personal vision 30, 36, 52, 181
personality 129, 156
personhood 105, 177, 184
phronesis (definition) 178-179
Picasso 62, 88
Pinpointing Professional Judgements 108
portfolio xv, 72, 136, 147, 158
    anonymising 72, 123, 164, 171
    uploaded 72, 136
postgraduate medical education 11, 14-15, 26, 45, 50, 128, 145, 166
practical reasoning 83-84, 104, 177-178, 181, 191
praxis 36, 38-40, 178-179, 188
preparation for teaching 145
principles and components of TRP 49, 51
Product Professional Judgement 63, 100, 102-103, 114, 206
Professional conversation 41, 123, 134-135, 152-153
professional identity 67, 119, 172, 176
professional values 70, 83, 138
professionalism 2, 13, 15-18, 20-21, 31, 49, 52, 54-55, 58, 61, 82, 119, 153, 163-165
protocols xvi, 16-18, 35, 42, 82, 84, 123, 133

qualities of clinical thinking 67, 105-106
qualities of professionalism 31, 36
Quality and wisdom 57
Quality Assurance 144

Rainbow writing colours 60, 64, 76, 195
Rainbow Writing 64, 67, 75-76, 95, 120, 152, 158, 164 207
reclaiming our professionalism 163
Reflection in healthcare more generally 34
reflection in practice 23
reflection on practice 23, 27, 29, 34, 37-39, 167, 178
reflective case evidence 118-119, 172
reflective cycle 40, 45
Reflective tradition 43
research 1-2, 5, 33-34, 43, 49, 51, 55, 57, 70, 163, 165, 167
ResPublica Trust 18, 20

safety and quality 119, 171-172
seeing with the heart 175-176
seeing the heart as teaching the mind 192
Science and Charity' 62, 88
Self-evaluation questions 160
Self-interested judgement 106
Self-knowledge 36, 167, 173, 189
self-serving interest groups 20
sensitivity 15, 132, 181, 189
servants of society 3
serving 3, 6, 20, 46, 49
sharing 117, 120, 134, 164-165, 167, 169-170, 172, 176
SPA time 70
spiritual practice 175-176, 182, 184-185, 192
    a conversation 23, 175, 178, 185
spiritual wisdom 4, 175, 177-179, 181 185, 191
spirituality 21, 129, 175-177, 179-180, 182, 185
Starting with your learner 125, 128
Studying the learner 129
Summarising the results 54, 117
Swampy lowlands 42
systematic critical enquiry 28

Talking and writing 9, 32, 125, 134, 141, 154
The exploratory Invisibles 56, 60, 63, 99
The interrogative Invisibles 52
The Narrative Invisibles 52, 55-56, 61, 75-78

The therapeutic relationship 56, 59, 62, 64, 88-89,
The wisdom of the heart 164, 175, 177, 181-182, 191-192
Thinking like a teacher 126, 141
Tradition 5, 9, 13, 31, 33, 38, 44-45, 123, 163
trust xvii, 4, 11, 19, 91, 119-120, 170-172, 183

Underpinning thinking 61, 78, 107, 111

Values xvii, 14, 23-25, 28, 31, 35-37, 46, 58, 61, 70, 80-81, 83, 118, 130-131, 133, 138, 143, 146, 155, 157, 159, 175, 177, 179-180, 182-185
virtue 18-19, 31, 36, 38, 80, 89, 178-179
voice
    refining your first draft 75, 91

wants and needs 20
wider perspective 51, 56, 83
wisdom of the heart 164, 175, 177, 181, 191-192
    the new heuristic 164, 178, 191
    with Aristotle 181-182
wise doctor 26, 62, 128
wise judgement 31, 105-107
worthwhile education 9, 23-24, 45, 126, 130, 139, 146, 158, 163
writing
    digitally 69, 71
    for learning 125, 134, 156

www.ingramcontent.com/pod-product-compliance
Ingram Content Group UK Ltd.
Pitfield, Milton Keynes, MK11 3LW, UK
UKHW062045180426
11947UKWH00030B/2052